LOOKGOOD
&FEELGOOD

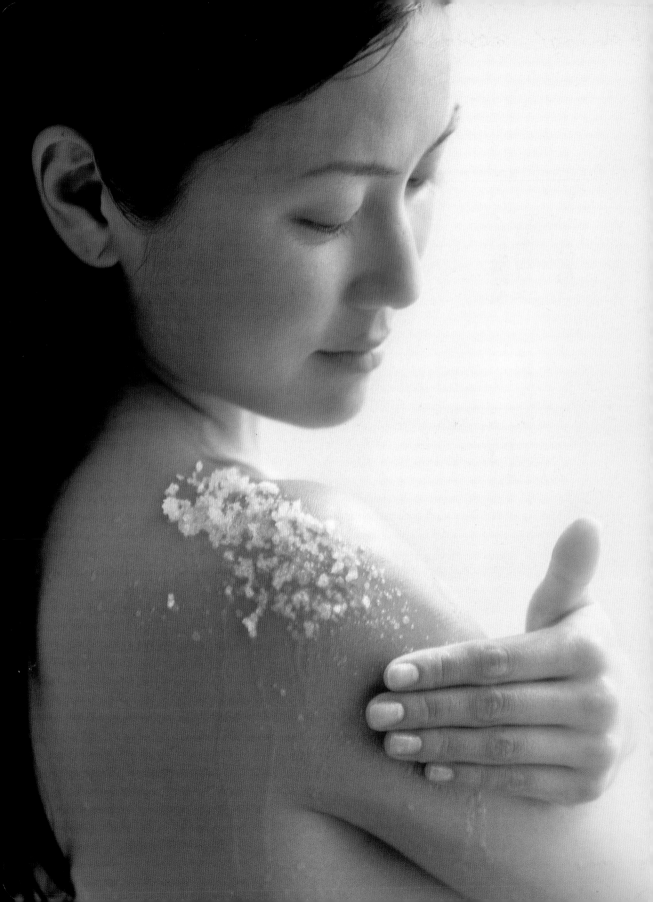

LOOKGOOD
FEELGOOD

206 beauty and fitness secrets

weldon**owen**

Contents

Introduction and Taking Care

de-stress

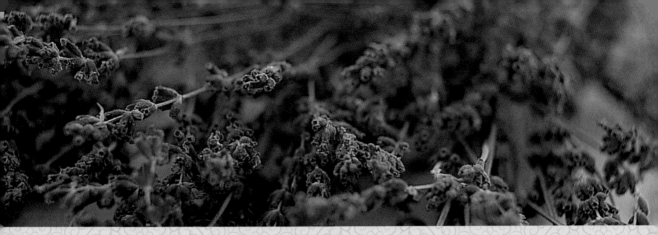

refresh

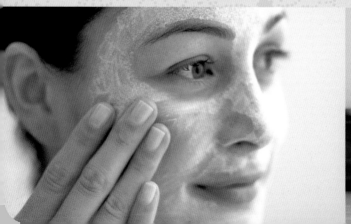

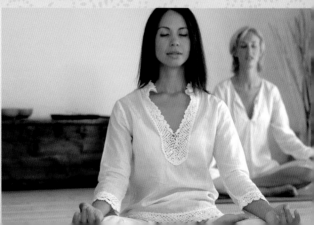

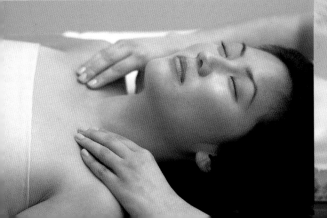

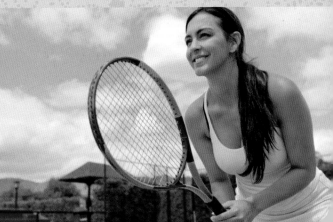

energize

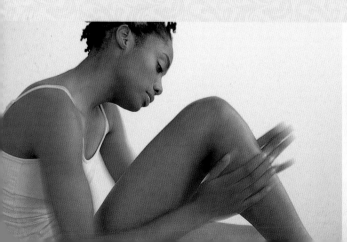

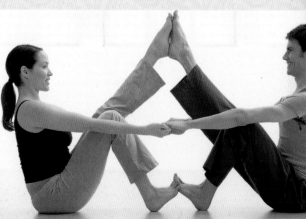

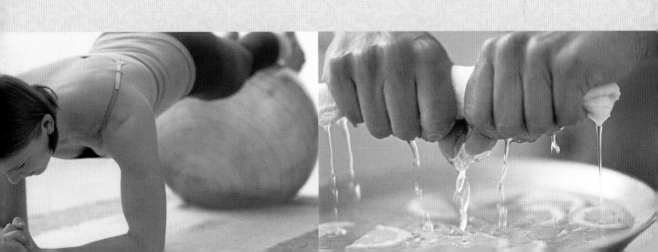

indulge

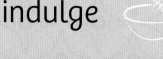

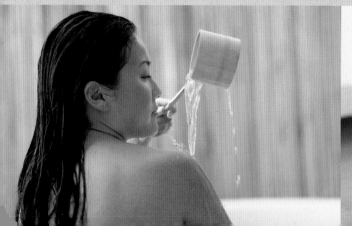

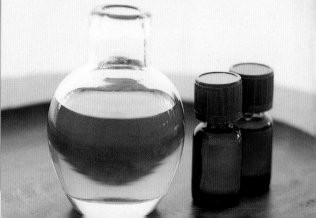

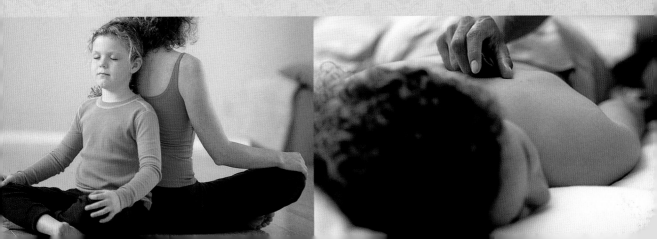

Introduction

Health, well-being, beauty, calm . . . these are all things we aspire to have in our lives.
Who wouldn't want to live a stress-free, centered life—and, just coincidentally, have
gorgeous hair, glowing skin, and a shapely figure? We know these things are important
and rewarding but so often in the rush of everyday life, we put off caring for ourselves.
Who has time for meditation, exercise, or luxury? The answer is that everyone can have
the time. That's where this book comes in.

In the pages that follow, you'll find hundreds of simple, imaginative, and practical ideas
for enhancing your health, outlook, and appearance. Drawn from a variety of fields,
including everything from aromatherapy and yoga, to massage and nutrition, these
ideas are organized thematically to help you attain specific benefits, such as renewed
energy, a stronger body, blissful relaxation, or a little well-earned pampering. The approach
is holistic—the needs of the body, mind, and spirit are all addressed—and the activities, all
contributed by experts in their fields, combine the best of time-honored, traditional
disciplines with the latest scientific findings.

The activities described here will give you a taste of many treatments and traditions
including skin care, hair care, spa treatments, aromatherapy, massage, yoga, meditation,
breathing techniques, Pilates, tai chi, general fitness, and nutrition. The exercises are
designed for beginners, but the descriptions aren't meant to be treatises on the subject.
Rather, the intention is that these peeks into various disciplines and ideas will help you
identify some new fields that interest you and lead you to investigate them further.

Read *Look Good, Feel Good* from beginning to end, or just start by looking for the
chapters that most spark your interest—whether it's learning new ways to unwind, new
ways to prevent illness, or new reasons to treat yourself with a little more care. Read on
for brief synopses of the treatments and traditions covered.

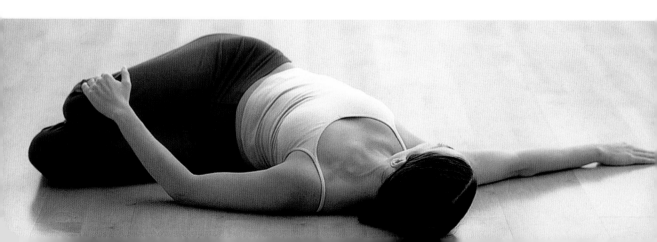

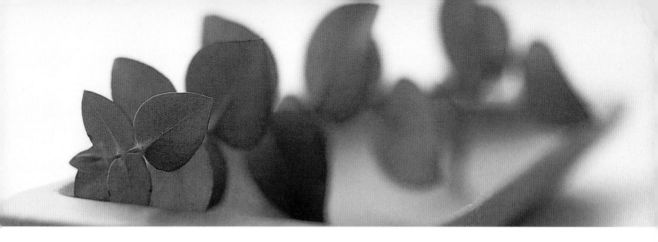

skin care, hair care, and beauty treatments

The world of beauty has long been the domain of women and has long been filled with all
sorts of wonderful (and sometimes not-so-wonderful) tips that are passed from mother to
daughter, friend to friend, and beautician to client. Throughout the 20th century, and even
today, some beauty products have become increasingly laden with chemicals and oriented
toward covering, rather than enhancing, our features. But these days, numerous simple,
natural products are also available to make you look and feel your best. The greatest beauty
secret of all? Many of the treatments are doable in just a few minutes in the privacy of your
home, as you'll see in the suggestions we offer in the following pages.

aromatherapy

The use of essential oils (oils distilled from aromatic plants) to promote physical, emotional,
and spiritual health dates back at least 6,000 years. Today, essential oils are used in a number
of ways—in massage oils and body lotions, dispersed in the bath, and diffused in the air.
Available in health and beauty stores, as well as on the Internet, essential oils are used to treat
a range of maladies and conditions, including stress, depression, headaches, anxiety, menstrual
discomfort, and skin problems. While some say that anything that smells good will make you
feel good, recent scientific research has shown that aromatherapy truly has health benefits.

massage

In today's fast-paced, individualistic world, one crucial lesson is often forgotten:
Humans need touch, and touch is a powerful healer. Indeed, for thousands of years, many
cultures have practiced some form of massage with the aim of easing physical, mental, and
spiritual ailments. That's not simply the stuff of folklore—research shows us again and again
that touch can help reduce stress hormones, alleviate depression, boost the immune system,
and diminish pain. And effective massages don't have to come only from certified massage
therapists. Simple massages—like those we've chosen here—can also be exchanged at home
between lovers, friends, and family members, as well as administered to oneself.

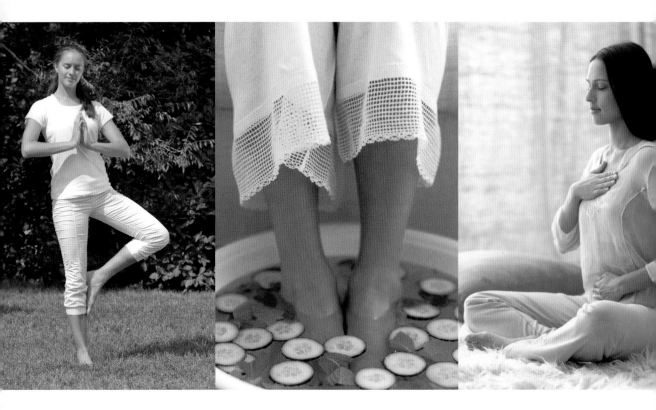

tai chi

An ancient martial art that originated in China, *tai chi* (pronounced tie-CHEE) is also known as Chinese shadow boxing. Now it is used as both a fighting and a healing technique, as well as a form of moving meditation. In Chinese, *tai* means "great" and *chi* means "energy," and the practice is all about experiencing, strengthening, and enhancing the flow of life energy in the body. Tai chi consists of a series of slow, graceful, and, ultimately, very powerful movements that involve the whole body and require intense mental focus. A sequence of tai chi movements is called a form, and if you practice these forms on a regular basis, they'll help you stay physically healthy, mentally sharp, and spiritually grounded. Some forms are difficult; the exercises we've included are simple enough for anyone to try at home.

general fitness

A strong body gives you the foundation for moving with confidence through the world. People who are fit tend to feel more capable and energetic; they also reduce their risks of getting some diseases, of becoming obese, and of falling and suffering physical injuries. We've chosen a variety of general fitness exercises to help you strengthen your body and enliven your workout routine.

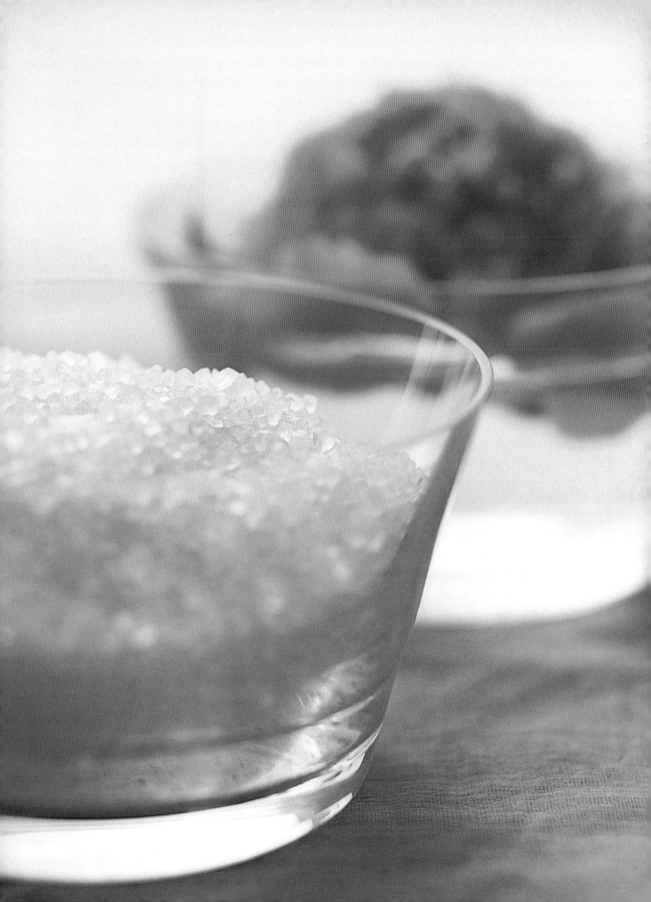

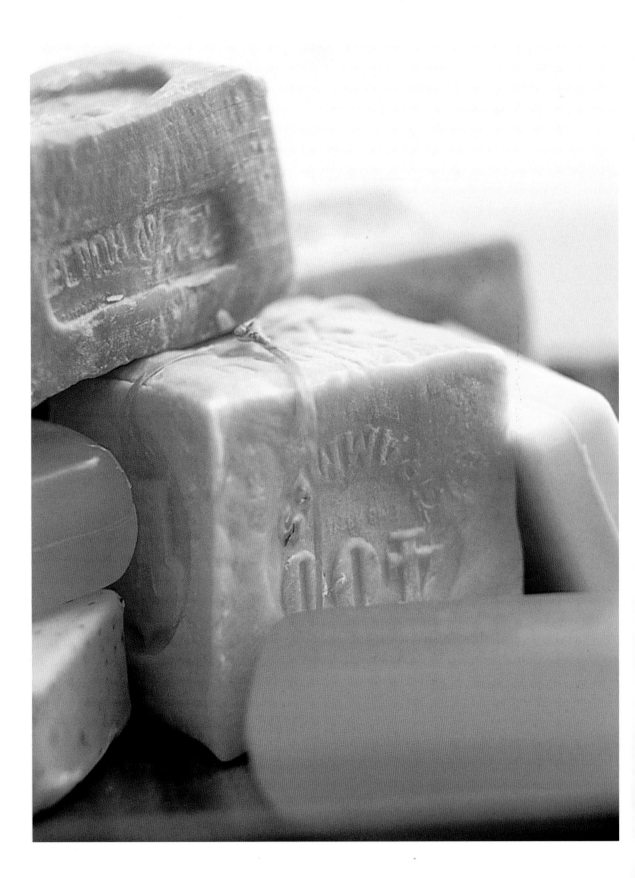

Taking Care

Some of the activities described in this book could be dangerous if performed incorrectly. When performing the physical exercises, for example, please take the time to read the text—don't just look at the pictures—and never push so hard that your body hurts. When you're practicing massage, it's important to remember not to massage directly on top of the spine or over varicose veins, open wounds, areas of intense pain, skin rashes, infections, or bruises. If you're pregnant, avoid exercises that impact the abdomen and those requiring deep work on your hands or feet. Pregnant women also shouldn't experiment with aromatherapy, and anyone using essential oils should read the instructions and warnings on the product labels before even opening the bottles. For instance, essential oils are almost never to be applied undiluted directly on the skin, and people with high blood pressure should avoid using stimulating oils. Be sure to perform patch tests of all beauty products to determine whether you might have an allergic reaction to the ingredients. If you're uncertain about the suitability of an exercise program or health-related practice, consult with your doctor or other health-care professional to determine whether it's right for you.

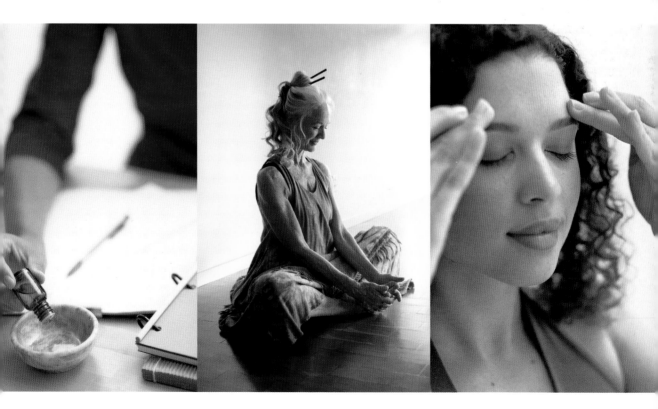

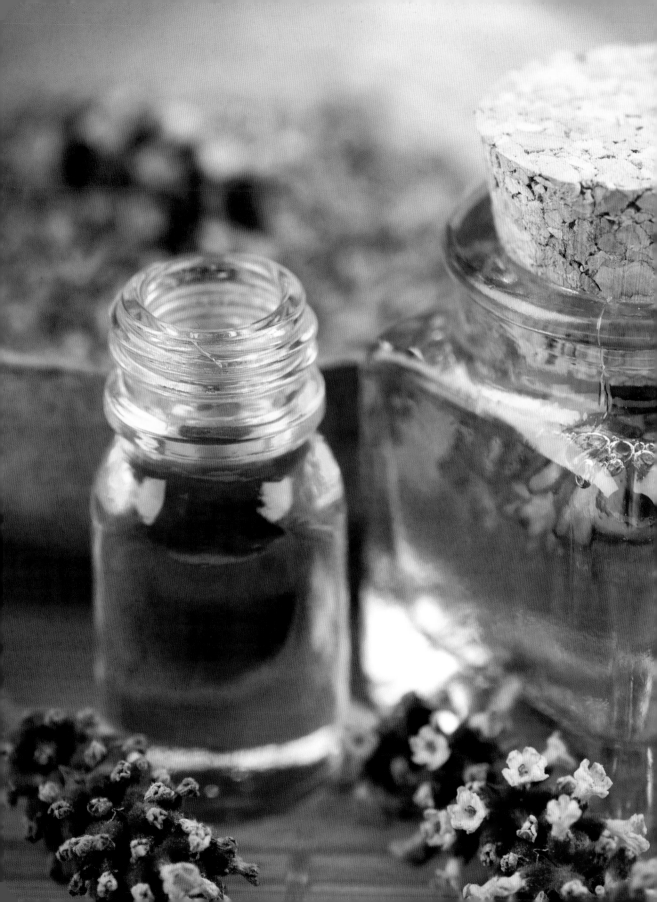

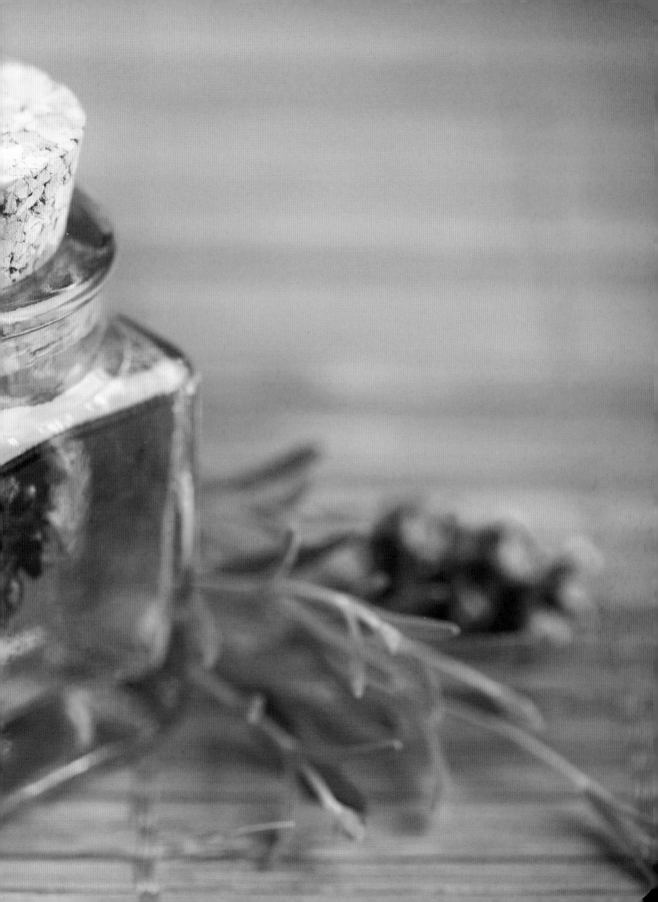

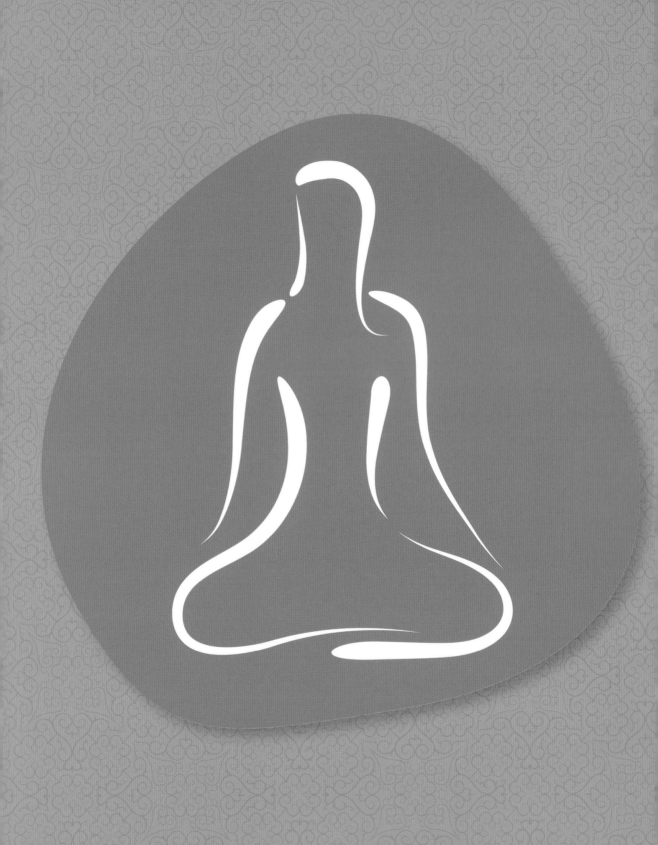

de-stress

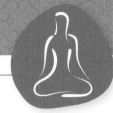

A hectic daily routine—never mind those spur-of-the-moment crises—can wreak havoc on your mind and body. Just as muscles need time to recover between strength-training sessions, your entire being needs time to relax amid the whirlwind of activities.

Taking the time to daydream, stretch, and observe the world around you can yield some amazing dividends. Your mind clears, your body recovers, and your spirit has the freedom to soar.

Remember that letting things go can be as important as getting them done. In fact, letting go is sometimes the best way to ensure that you are able to do your best. After all, a relaxed body moves more freely. A calm mind hears its muse more easily. And a tranquil heart can better be open to feeling love and happiness. ﾍ

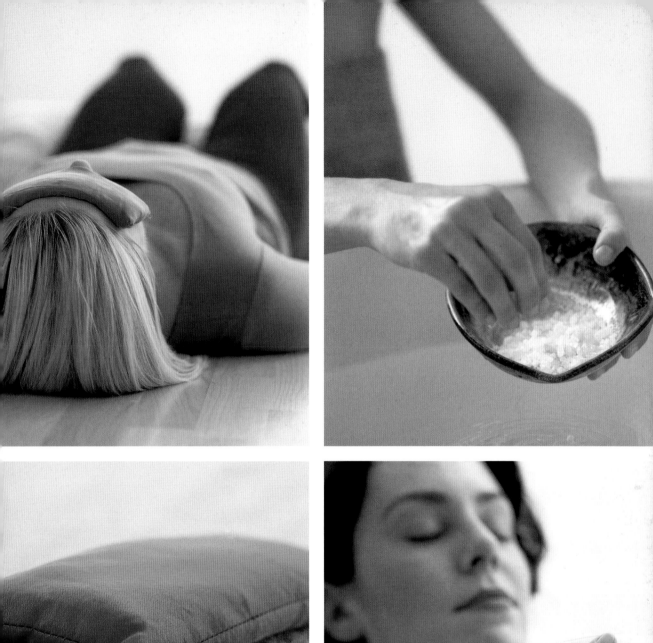
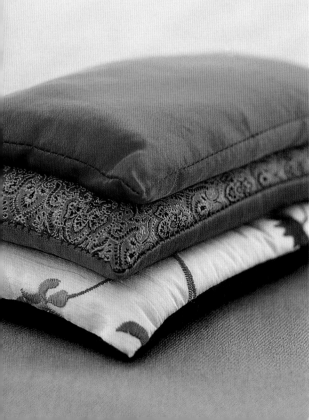
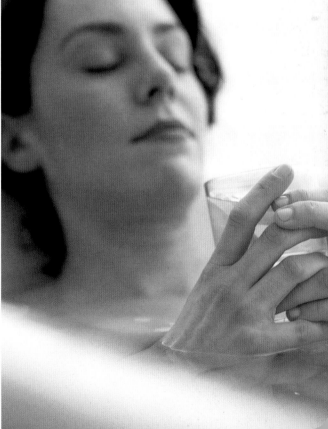

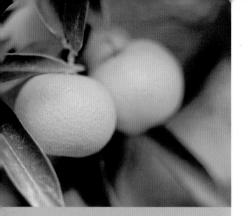

01

Use Bergamot to Energize

The use of essential oils (oils distilled from aromatic plants) to promote physical, emotional, and spiritual health dates back at least 6,000 years. Today, essential oils are used in a number of ways—in massage oils and body lotions, dispersed in the bath, and diffused in the air.

Bergamot's bright, citrusy flavor gives Earl Grey tea its distinctive taste. The fruit's essential oil, which is distilled from its peel, has been used for medicinal and skin-care purposes since Renaissance times. Bergamot's scent is extremely uplifting and soothing; aromatherapists recommend it for treating anxiety, anger, fear, and even mild depression.

02 Be Nice to Your Neck

After a hectic day, treat yourself to a scented, heated neck wrap or pillow to ease some of the tension and discomfort that builds up in your neck and shoulders. The heat also promotes an increased range of movement in your neck.

1 Purchase a heatable wrap or soft pillow that conforms well to the contours of your neck and is filled with rice and aromatic herbs. The weight of the rice puts subtle pressure on your muscles, helping to loosen them; the scent of the herbs is calming to frazzled nerves; and the heat helps melt away tension and soreness.

2 To enhance the relaxing effect of this treatment, you might want to sprinkle a few drops of essential oil onto your neck wrap or pillow. Pick a soothing scent that goes well with any herbs or other plants already contained in the wrap. For example, jasmine harmonizes with lavender, and chamomile complements rosemary. Bergamot is an especially soothing and reassuring scent that blends well with many other aromatic oils, including cypress, ginger, palmarosa, juniper, lemon, neroli, ylang-ylang, and geranium. If you're using a pure essential oil, be sure to mix it with a little carrier oil before sprinkling it on the pillow to avoid skin irritation.

3 Find a quiet spot to sit where you can lean back with your head supported, such as an upholstered, high-backed chair. Heat the pillow or wrap as directed by its manufacturer, and place it behind your neck, on top of your shoulders. Sit back and relax for about ten minutes, or until the pillow or wrap cools and your tension has faded away—at least until you face tomorrow's challenges.

03 Nod Your Neck to Let Stress Go

Stuck at your desk and stressed to the max? Try a little self-massage to unwind. Press your right thumb into the base of your skull near your right ear and nod your head three to six times. Inch your thumb across the ridge of your skull toward the spine, nodding at each spot. Repeat on the left side.

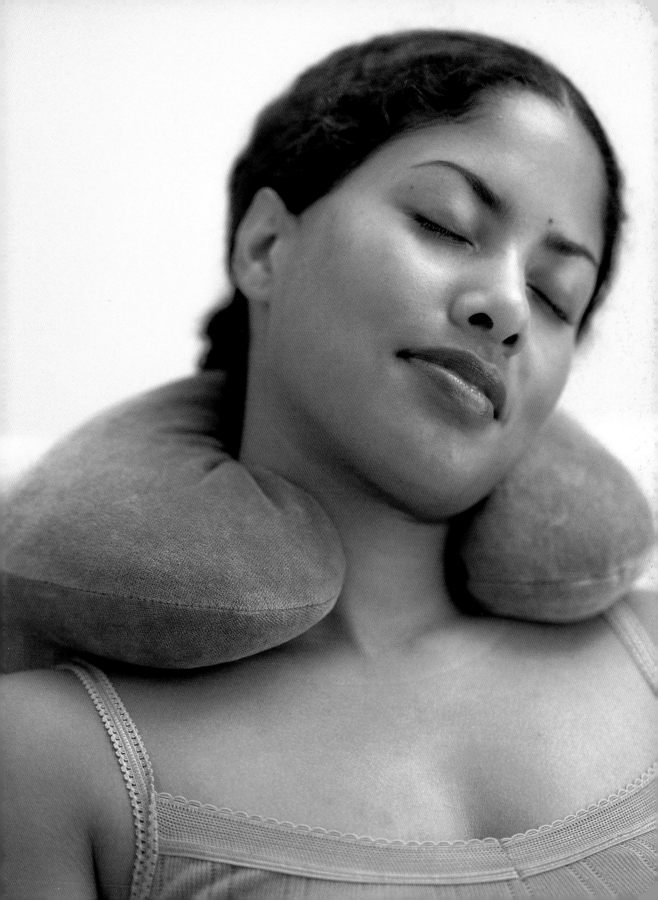

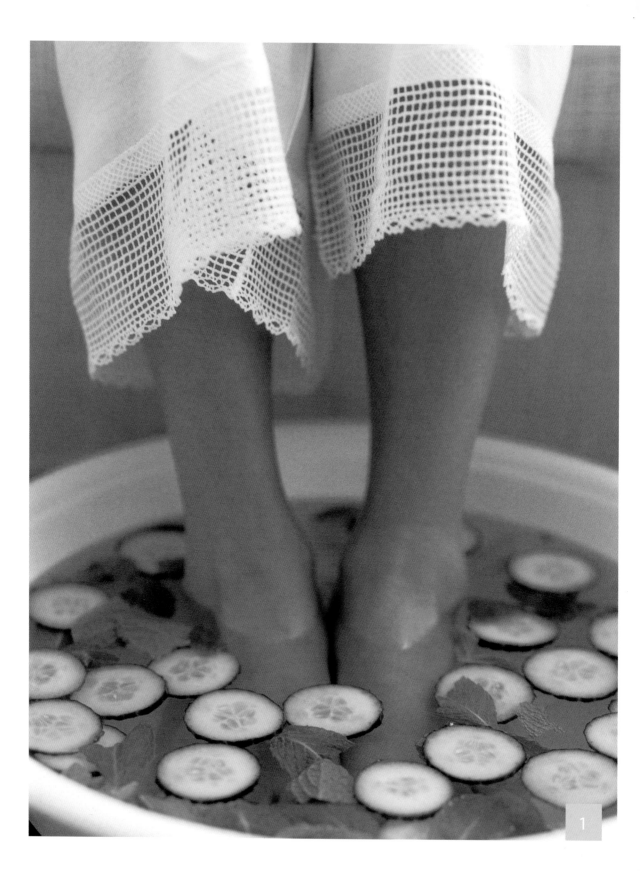

04 Give Tired Feet a Time-Out

When your feet are weary and ache after a long day, soak, roll, and massage your way to immediate relief with this series of soothing at-home spa treatments.

1 Fill a large bowl with cool water. Add six drops of tea tree essential oil and stir. Then add a couple dozen cucumber slices and a handful of torn fresh mint leaves. (Tea tree essential oil has antibacterial properties, cucumber acts as a mild astringent, and mint imparts a fresh scent.) Place the bowl at the foot of your favorite chair and ease your feet into the water. Relax, and soak your feet for about 15 minutes.

2 After your soak, dry your feet off and sit in a chair. Place one foot on a wooden foot roller, and move it forward and back, varying the speed and pressure. Massage for five to ten minutes, then switch feet.

3 Give your feet a massage. Using a generous amount of lotion, balm, or massage oil with an appealing scent, vigorously massage one foot, rubbing briskly back and forth. Then, with your hands wrapped around the arch of your foot, squeeze your hands together firmly and glide them toward your toes. This action increases circulation and helps remove toxins. Repeat on your other foot.

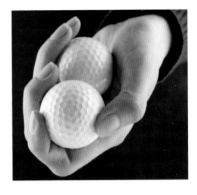

Try At-Home Reflexology

When you use a wooden foot roller, you're actually doing much more than simply soothing your aching feet. In fact, the foot roller is designed to activate the reflexology zones of the soles of your feet. For a DIY version, knot a few golf balls in a sock to give yourself a quickie foot massage.

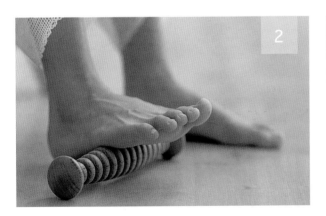

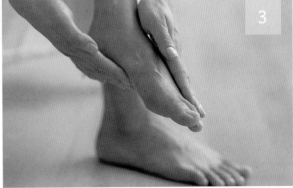

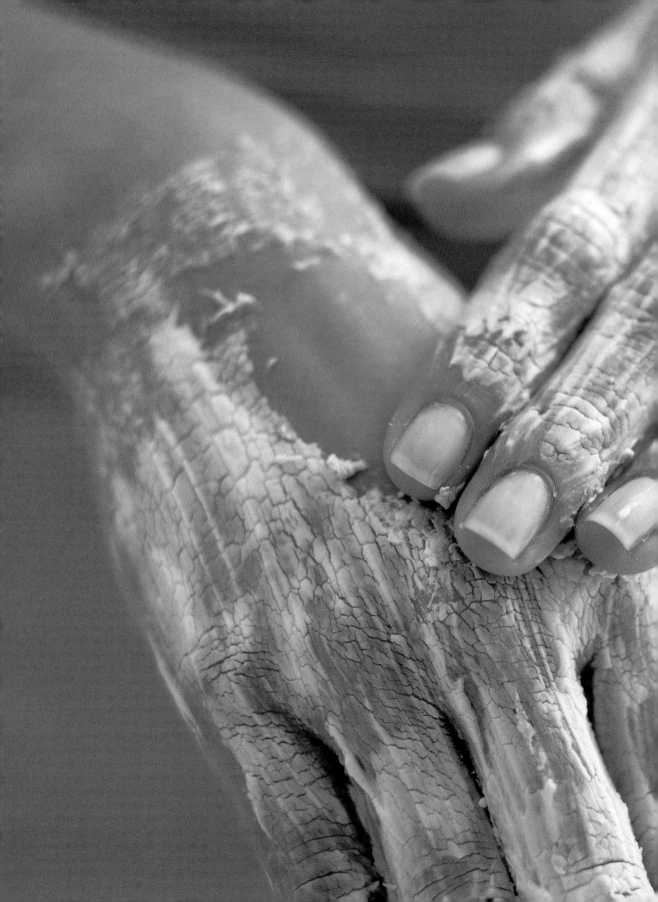

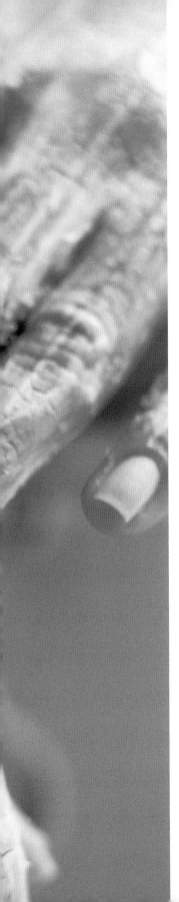

05 Soften Your Hands with Sweet Almond Oil

We often forget how hard our hands work until we notice they are dry or rough. Pampering hands from time to time makes them look and feel better. Give your hands a well-deserved scrub with products featuring sweet almond oil, a light and delicately scented oil that promotes soft skin and flexible nails. A key ingredient in many massage and moisturizing lotions, sweet almond oil is ideal for dry, chapped, mature, or simply overworked hands because it contains essential fatty acids, which protect and replenish the skin and help keep nails healthy and supple.

06 Add Almond Oil to Your Grocery List

The sweet almond (the formal name for the common snack food) is a fruit. The flesh is hard, leathery, and dull green; it dries up when ripe, leaving a rough shell that contains the kernel that we both eat and use for oil. In addition to its virtues as a beauty aid, almond oil is a cholesterol-free salad and cooking oil filled with vitamin E, essential fatty acids, and heart-healthy monounsaturated fats. To preserve its delicate flavor, substitute cold-pressed almond oil for olive oil or nut oil, such as hazelnut or walnut, in salads and other cold dishes.

07 Improvise Gloves for Overnight Moisturizing

If your hands are dry, soften their skin while you sleep by applying sweet almond oil and slipping a pair of cotton socks over them. Other oils, such as vitamin E, jojoba, or olive oil, are also good choices, as is any rich hand cream. The socks intensify the effects of the moisturizer.

08 Exfoliate to Reveal Softer Hands

Give your hands some TLC by exfoliating, conditioning, and moisturizing them with products that contain sweet almond oil. This treatment—using an exfoliating scrub, nail balm, and hand cream—will nourish your skin, cuticles, and nails.

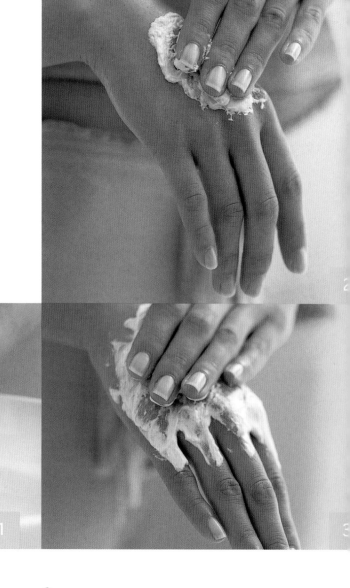

1 Fill a bowl or sink with warm water and wash your hands with a mild soap. Avoid using very hot water, as it can further dry your skin. Wash your hands purposefully. Take a few minutes to massage them by pressing your thumbs into your palms, and gently squeeze each finger, working from the bottom to the top of each. Then rinse and dry your hands.

2 Once your hands are completely dry, spread an exfoliating scrub containing sweet almond oil (see recipe at top right) on the back of each hand.

3 Put a thick, even layer of the scrub on your hands and over the entire length of your fingers. Then allow the scrub to dry for about ten minutes.

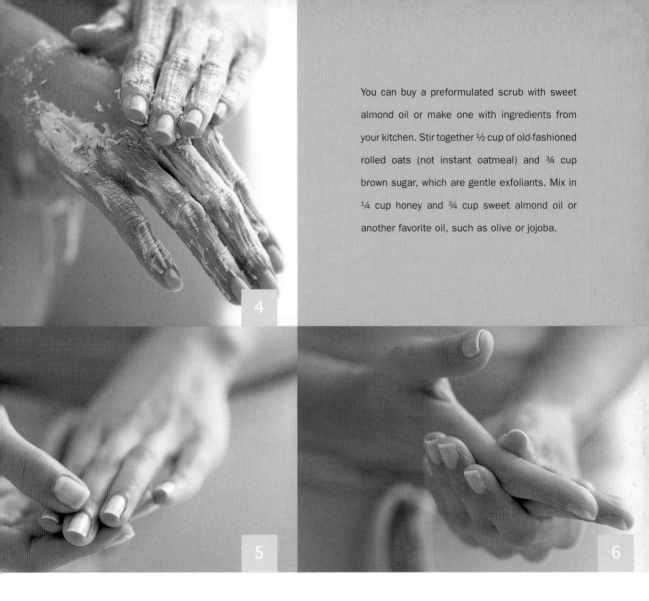

You can buy a preformulated scrub with sweet almond oil or make one with ingredients from your kitchen. Stir together ½ cup of old-fashioned rolled oats (not instant oatmeal) and ¾ cup brown sugar, which are gentle exfoliants. Mix in ¼ cup honey and ¾ cup sweet almond oil or another favorite oil, such as olive or jojoba.

4 When the scrub has a chalky consistency, it's dry and ready to remove. Simply rub your hands together until most of the product flakes off. Or use a clean, dry washcloth to thoroughly brush the scrub off your hands.

5 Rinse your hands in warm (not hot) water and dry them thoroughly.

6 Now condition your fingernails and cuticles with sweet almond oil nail balm. Massage a generous amount onto the surface of each nail and into the cuticle. When the nail balm has been absorbed, apply a highly emollient sweet almond cream liberally over both hands.

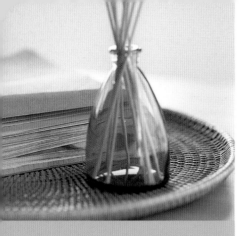

09

Use a Reed Diffuser

If you prefer not to use electricity or a candle to diffuse aromas, opt for a reed diffuser. Essential oil is stored in a container and is drawn upward through slender bamboo reeds, providing an ongoing release of beneficial scents in the room.

10 Uplift with Aromatherapy

When you're feeling stressed, anxious, or sad, help brighten your mood by infusing your environment with the soothing scents of calming, peaceful, and uplifting essential oils.

Release the aromas of pure essential oils with a diffuser. This pleasing and effective method creates a mood-altering ambiance and unleashes the various therapeutic properties of the oils. Many types of aromatherapy diffusers are available—clay, glass, ceramic, and metal—and some are as decorative as they are efficient.

Diffusers are designed with dishes or wells in which to place the essential oils, which are usually diluted with water or a carrier oil (follow the manufacturer's instructions on the proper use of your particular model). Many are warmed by small candles, but there are also electric diffusers that circulate cool air. If you use candles in your diffuser, make sure they're unscented, so they don't interfere with the aroma produced by the oils you've selected.

11 Try Different Oils for Different Effects

Essential oils are used to treat a range of conditions. To help relieve tension, anxiety, or sadness, try diffusing oils such as ylang-ylang, lavender, and rose. Neroli, bergamot, geranium, clary sage, and palmarosa are also considered calming and help restore a sense of balance and optimism—a useful air freshener, indeed.

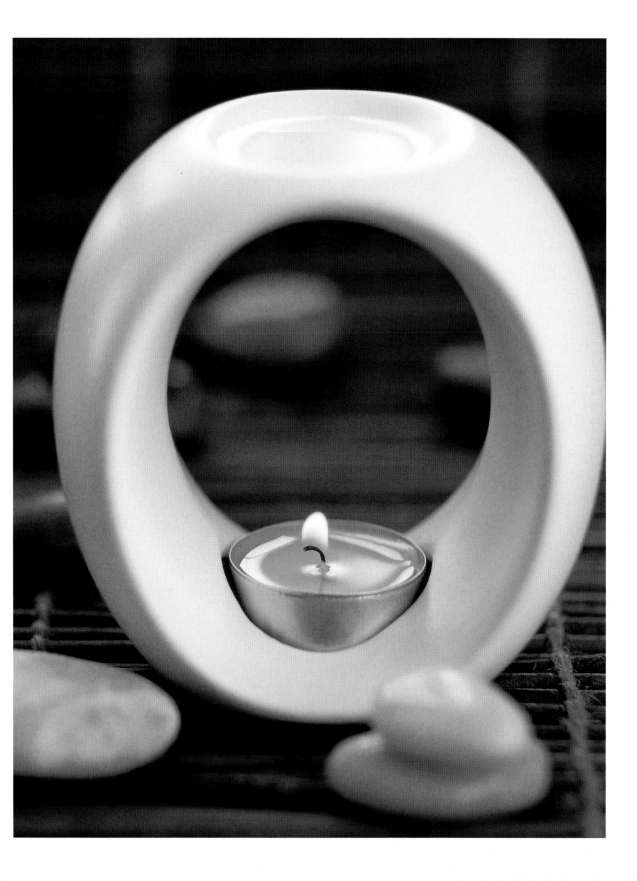

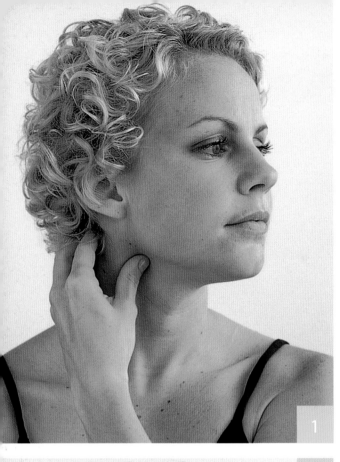

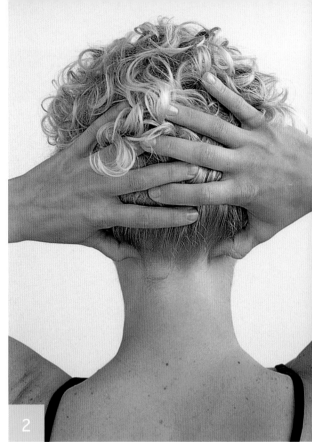

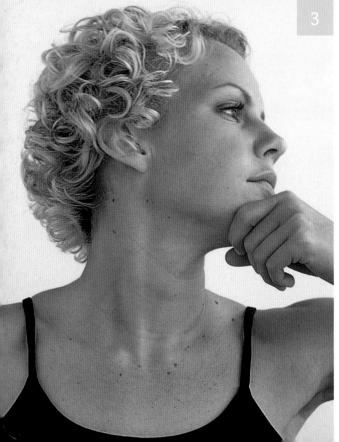

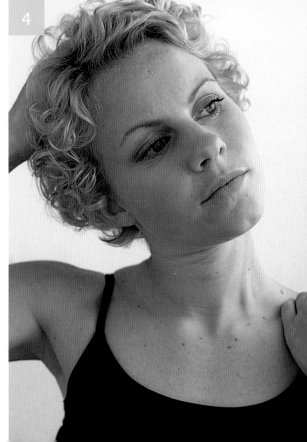

1

2

3

4

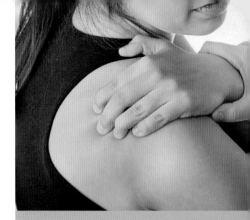

12 Knead the Knots Out of Your Neck

Even if no one is around to lend a helping hand, you can find welcome neck relief with this series of do-it-yourself rubs and stretches.

1 Turn your head to the side to find your sternocleidomastoid muscle (for obvious reasons, usually just referred to as the SCM). The SCM starts on the breastbone and collarbone, crosses the neck at an angle, and attaches to the base of the skull behind the ear. Press in with your thumb and grasp the bottom of the SCM from behind. Hold using firm pressure while you slowly turn your head from side to side three times. Then repeat in a new spot one inch higher. Work both sides of your neck from bottom to top.

2 Now turn your attention to the back of your head. Press in firmly with your thumbs at the base of your skull and move them in tight, firm circles. Begin on either side of the spine and work outward along the base of your skull toward the ears. If you encounter sore points, stop and press firmly on each as you take three deep breaths.

3 Grasp something stable, such as a tabletop, with your right hand and turn your head as far to the left as is comfortable, sitting or standing up tall. Stretch your neck muscles by gently guiding your chin farther to the left with your left hand. Hold the stretch for three deep breaths. Gently release and repeat on the other side.

4 Place your left hand on your left shoulder. With your right hand, gently guide your head down toward your right shoulder. Breathe in and out slowly, feeling your neck muscles gradually lengthen over the span of three breaths. Bring your head slowly back to center. Repeat on the other side. You can do this stretch a number of times, holding your head at different angles to isolate various muscles.

13 Don't Fight It

Part of the reason your neck and shoulders ache when you're under stress is the fight-or-flight mode that the body automatically assumes when exposed to a threat, whether a hungry tiger or a peevish boss! When this self-preservation mechanism kicks in, the shoulders hunch upward and the neck instinctively cocks the head forward. Consciously take a moment to release that defensive posture when you're in the middle of a rough day.

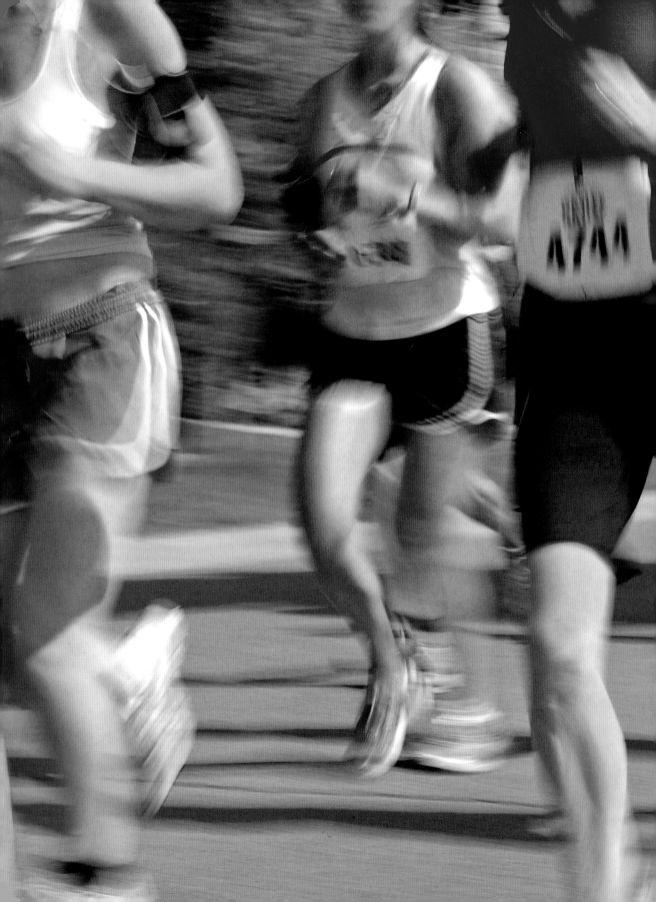

14 Move to a Better Mood

Move it *and* lose it—stress, that is. Regular cardiovascular workouts—defined as vigorous exercise that works up a sweat—have physical and emotional benefits. Cardio exercise has been shown to reduce stress, ease anxiety, and elevate mood. Turns out the stress link is both neurochemical and behavioral. When you exercise, levels of hormones that trigger and exacerbate stress, such as adrenaline and cortisol, decrease. Meanwhile, your brain releases pain-killing, mood-lifting endorphins. The effect also has a behavioral link. Call it a positive-feedback loop: You work out on a regular basis, and before long you start feeling stronger. Your skin glows. You sleep more soundly. You're alert during the day. Those things are mood-boosting, too, so you're motivated to lace up your shoes for another workout. Put simply, you feel good when you exercise—and we all naturally gravitate toward what makes us feel, well, good.

The key is finding the stress-busting workout that works for you. Cardio doesn't have to mean pounding out miles on a treadmill. In fact, you may not get the same mood-boosting effect if you don't enjoy the workout you choose. Your cardio outlet can be soccer or a belly-dancing class (team sports and classes are mood-boosters if you enjoy the camaraderie), a hike or a jump-rope session. Aim for 30 minutes (or more) of heart-pumping exercise five days a week. It counts if you split that into smaller time segments—taking the stairs, walking from the far end of the parking lot, doing an exercise podcast—it all adds up!

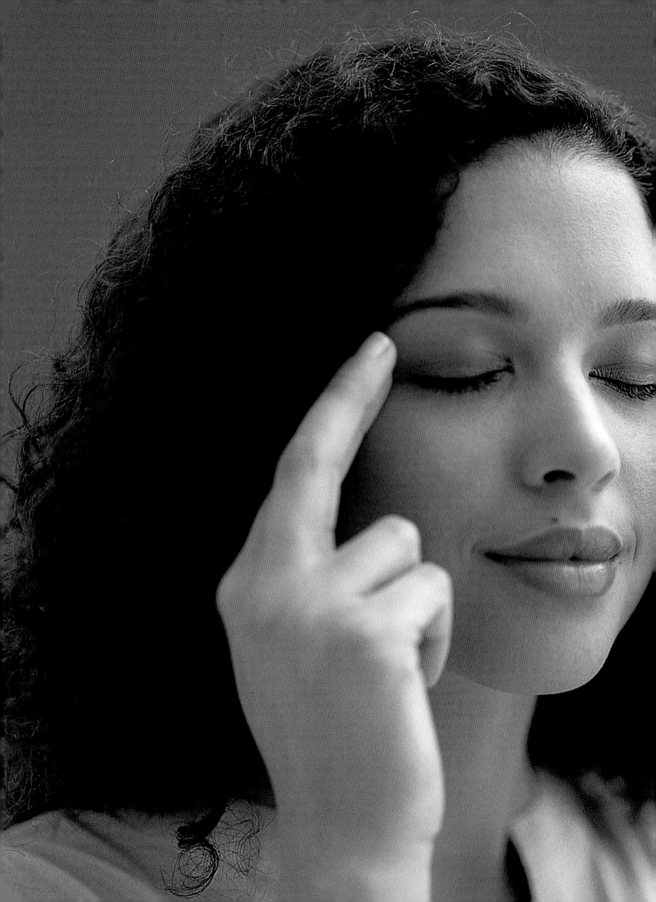

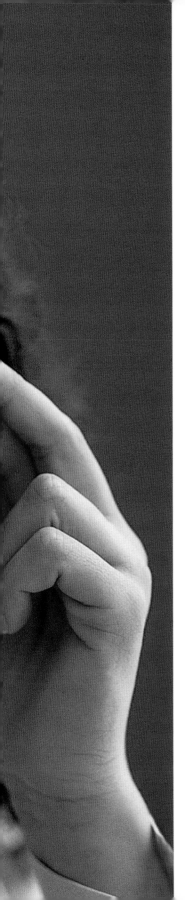

15 Find Relief for Weary Eyes

Staring at computer screens, reading small print, and frowning because you're concentrating (or just plain stressed) can wreak havoc on your eyes. Some people get headaches, some suffer from irritated eyes, and others find their vision actually starts to blur.

The trick is having the discipline to stop and take frequent breaks when you're overworking your eyes. Even just closing your eyes or looking out in the distance for a moment can help.

For some quick relief, try the easy-to-do self-massage and focusing exercises on the following pages. They are designed to help dispel headaches, soothe strained eye muscles, and relieve pent-up tension in the eyes—and throughout the rest of the body.

16 Relieve Tension with Your Fingertips

To help relieve facial tension, apply gentle fingertip pressure in circles on your temples, cheekbones, and chin. Start at your temples. With relaxed hands, gently circle up and back with your middle fingers pressed into the indented areas at the outside edges of your eyebrows. Breathe deeply and continue circling for three full breaths.

Next, massage your cheekbones. Starting at the sides of your nostrils, gently press in circles with your middle fingers. Circle your fingertips spot by spot along the contours of the bottom of your cheekbones toward your ears. Move your fingertips down to your chin. Placing your middle fingers between your lower lip and chin, press firmly and circle with your fingertips, moving outward and upward along the jawline and into the jaw muscles.

17 Relax Eye Muscles

Drawing upon massage, Eastern medicine, and yoga, these self-massage and focusing exercises help relax your eye muscles, bring more oxygen to your eyes, and activate energy meridians (the channels of energy that healers believe run through the body).

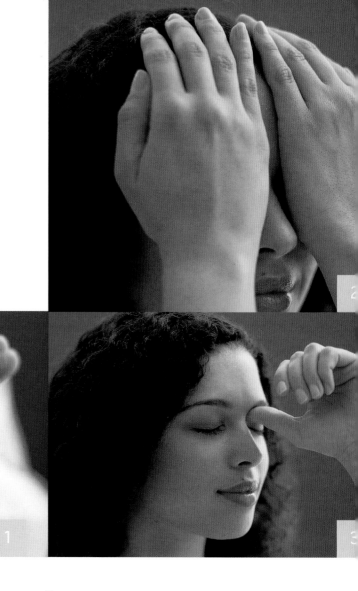

1 To practice eye palming, first wash your hands, then rub them together to warm them.

2 Cup your palms over closed eyes and rest your fingers over your forehead. Apply as much pressure to your eyes as feels comfortable. Breathe deeply. Hold this position for several minutes. (Note: Don't do eye palming if you're wearing contacts.)

3 Close your eyes and press your thumb into the point just beneath your left eyebrow and by the bridge of your nose. Press gently upward (be careful: this spot can be sore) for about a minute while breathing deeply. Repeat with the other eye.

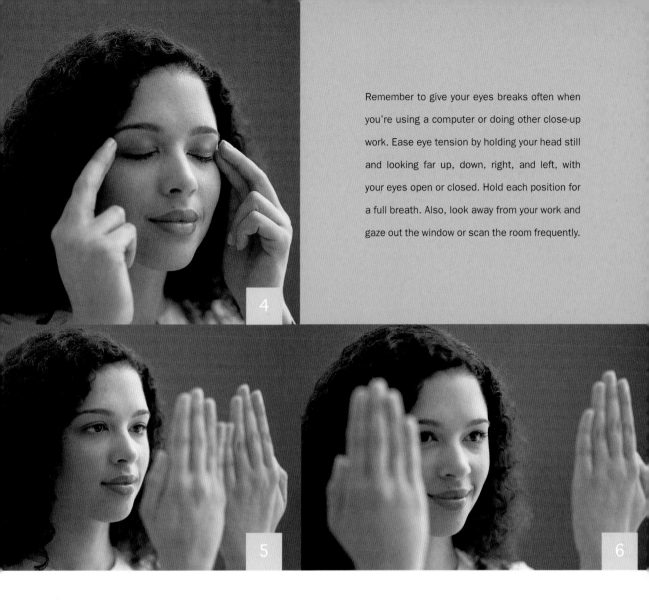

Remember to give your eyes breaks often when you're using a computer or doing other close-up work. Ease eye tension by holding your head still and looking far up, down, right, and left, with your eyes open or closed. Hold each position for a full breath. Also, look away from your work and gaze out the window or scan the room frequently.

4 Press two fingertips into the point at the outside edge of your eye. Lightly massage this area with a circular motion for a few minutes. In both Western and Eastern medical practices, this exercise is believed to improve blood circulation, which can relieve eye tension.

5 To give your eyes a break from constantly focusing on nearby objects, hold your hands about 12 inches in front of your face, with palms in and fingers together, pointing straight up.

6 As you inhale deeply, move your hands apart and look out at a distant spot. Now exhale and bring your hands together again, readjusting your focus to look at your palms. Repeat, alternating between hand positions (and focal points) for two to three minutes.

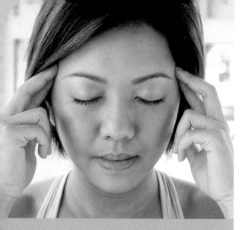

18
Stave Off Headaches

To help prevent headaches, the American Headache Society recommends you practice "headache hygiene":

- Go to sleep and wake up at the same time each day.

- Practice aerobic exercise for at least 30 minutes three times a week.

- Eat a good breakfast, and follow up with regular meals throughout the day.

- De-stress.

- Identify and avoid dietary triggers—foods that cause headaches.

19 Clear Your Head

When stress or fatigue leaves you unable to think straight, these simple moves increase the blood supply to your head, noticeably improving concentration and clarity.

1 With a rubber-bristled brush, brush your hair back from your hairline with long, firm strokes, moving all the way across your head. Next, hang your head upside down and brush your hair from your neckline to the crown of your head. Repeat both steps five times.

2 Using the pads of your fingertips, scrub slowly and deeply through your hair, all over your scalp. Begin at your forehead and work back over the crown of your head and down to the nape of your neck. After you've massaged your head for a few minutes, you may feel a tingling or pulsing sensation—a sign of increased blood flow, with its burst of brain-stimulating oxygen.

3 Now place your hands on both sides of your head, with the heels of your palms resting on your temples. Gently press your temples for five seconds, then release and glide your hands up to the crown of your head. Repeat the pressing and gliding sequence, varying both the amount of pressure and the speed of your strokes, until you can feel the tension in your head start to ease.

4 Finish your massage by slowly running your fingers through your hair, gently removing any tangles. Then, using light pressure, scratch your scalp with your fingernails, moving from your forehead to the nape of your neck; repeat three times. Each time, increase the pressure slightly. Finally, release any remaining scalp tension by gathering a handful of your hair together and pulling it gently downward. Hold the hair for three seconds before releasing, then move on to another handful of hair. Be sure to gently pull and release all your hair so your entire scalp benefits from the tension relief.

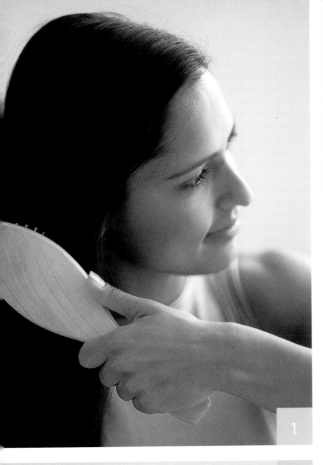

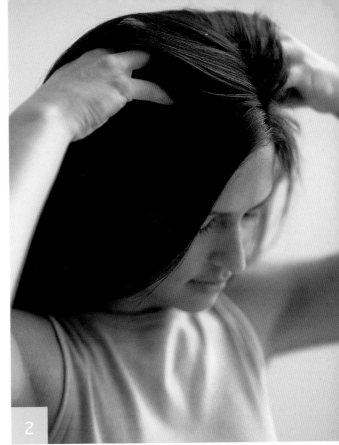

1

2

3

4

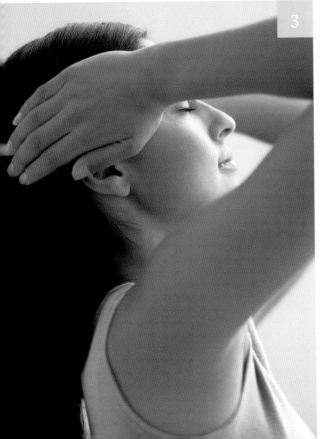

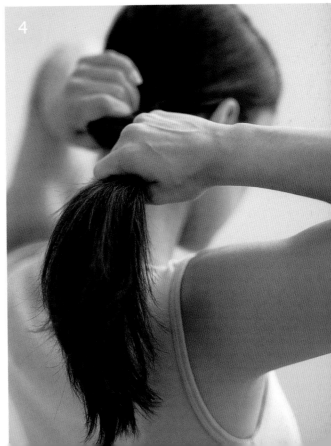

20 Curl Up to Soothe a Sore Back

This simple yoga stretch can ease a tense back and help you increase the range of motion in your back and hips. Lie on your back, bring your knees to your chest, and wrap your arms around your legs. Inhale deeply and hold your breath as you lift your chest toward your knees. Then rock gently, either from side to side or from head to hips, using the weight of your body to massage your back. When you're ready to exhale, release your breath all at once through your mouth and, at the same time, stretch out your limbs on the floor. Relax for a minute or two, then repeat.

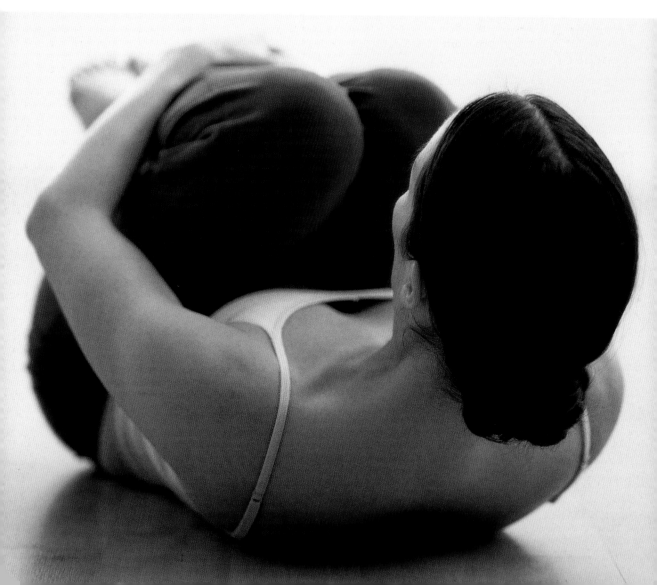

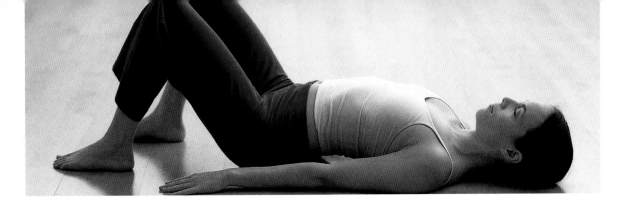

21 Tilt Your Pelvis

The pelvic tilt feels good on its own, and it is used in many yoga poses—as well as other forms of exercise—to protect the lower back from strain by strengthening core muscles. To assume this soothing pose, lie on your back on a comfortable surface with your knees bent and your feet on the floor hip-width apart. Rest your arms on the floor alongside your body. Inhale, arching your lower back and pressing your tailbone down. Then exhale, flattening your lower back down to the floor and pressing your tailbone upward. Continue this pattern for four to ten breaths, arching your back with each inhalation and flattening your back with each exhalation.

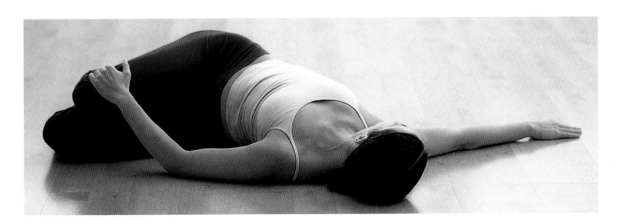

22 Try a Spinal Twist

Lying on your back, bring your legs together with your knees bent and extend your arms out from your shoulders along the floor with your palms down. Lower your bent legs toward the floor to your left, keeping your right shoulder grounded. If your knees don't reach the ground, you can put a folded blanket, rolled towel, or firm pillow under them for support. Gaze upward or, if you can do so comfortably, to your right. If you like, you can place your left hand on your knees to guide your legs down gently. Hold for ten breaths, and inhale as you bring your legs back to center, then repeat on your right side.

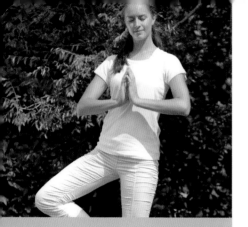

23
Balance Blindly

To make any standing yoga pose more challenging, try doing it with your eyes closed. It's trickier than you might think to maintain your balance when you lose your point of visual reference.

24 Achieve Better Balance with Mountain Pose

Balancing yoga poses help you better understand the interplay between movement and stillness. They also can improve your posture.

Start with the basic Mountain pose (see the photo at right): Stand with your feet together and your arms relaxed at your sides to form a long, straight line with your body. Tighten your quadriceps (the muscles on the front of your thighs) to help stabilize your knees and prevent them from locking. Keep your chin up and head facing forward. Release your shoulder blades so they are down and loose, keeping your collarbones lifted and wide. Relax the muscles of your face and throat. Challenge your balancing skills by closing your eyes. Hold for several breaths, visualizing the steadiness of a mountain.

Praying Mountain is a variation on this pose. Stand as before, tall and straight with your feet together. Instead of resting your arms by your sides, hold your hands in the prayer position (palms pressed together, fingers pointing up) and bring them up to chest level. Distribute your weight evenly on both feet, tighten your quadriceps, keep your shoulders dropped, and stand tall. Hold for several breaths.

25 Locate Your Equilibrium

To help maintain your balance, fix your gaze on a point at or just below eye level in front of you. Visualize a triangle of stability being created between three points: your eyes, the chosen point of focus, and your center of gravity (just below your navel). Learning to balance this way will help you achieve physical and mental equilibrium. Don't push yourself too hard on this notion, though. If you're having trouble balancing, practice poses near or against a wall. As your body and mind strengthen, you'll be able to give up the external support.

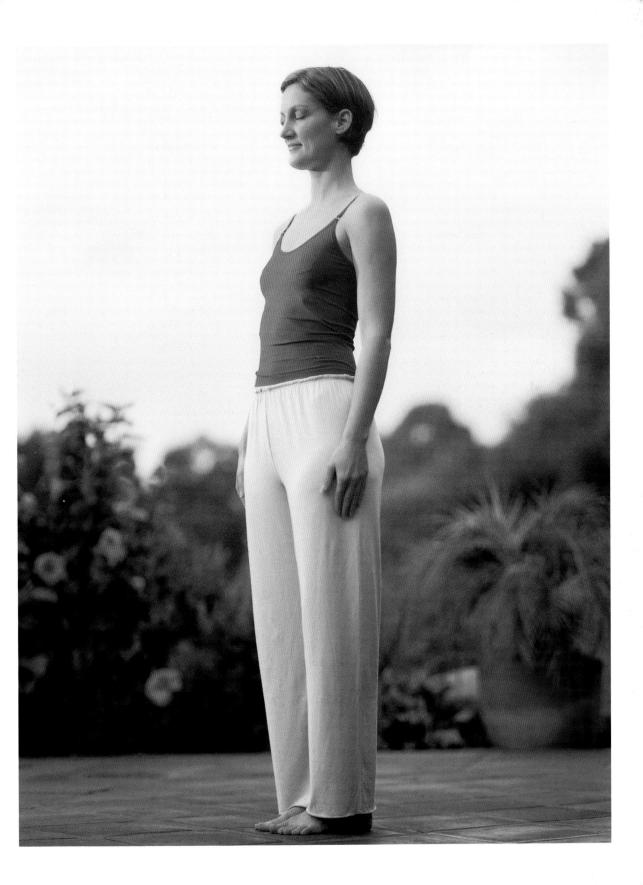

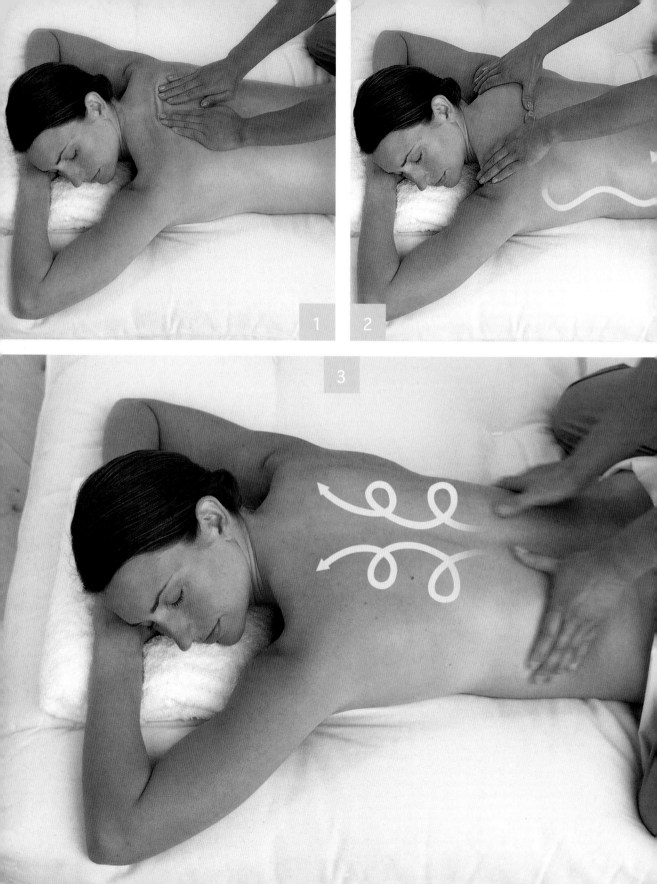

26 Get a Back-Friendly Massage

Whether coping with aches and pains or just aiming for a little overall relaxation, these techniques help relax the often tense and sore muscles of the back. Ask a friend to follow these simple massage steps:

1 After warming some massage oil in your hands (see the recipe at right), glide them up the thick muscles alongside her spine. Press firmly with your fingertips and palms, and contour your hands to fit the shape of her back as you glide. At the base of her neck, fan out your hands and stroke across the top and down the sides of her shoulders.

2 Curve your hands around her shoulders and pull down toward her ribs. Glide down the sides toward her hips, sweep your fingers under her waist, then lean back and gently pull toward you to stretch the muscles of her lower back. Repeat Steps 1 and 2 four more times.

3 Starting on the lower back, press your thumbs into the muscles on each side of her spine. Using firm pressure, circle your thumbs into the muscles as you gradually make your way up to her neck. Always be careful to press to the side of, never directly on, the spine. Then circle your thumbs into the muscles around the base of her neck and across her shoulders. Repeat three more times.

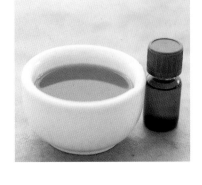

Massage Oil Blend

2 ounces carrier oil (such as sweet
　 almond, grape seed, or jojoba)
12 drops lavender essential oil
8 drops clary sage essential oil
5 drops ylang-ylang essential oil

27 Scratch Each Other's Backs

We've all heard the saying, "You scratch my back. I'll scratch yours." Well, in a different context, a good back-scratching can be quite soothing. Superficial nerves on the skin surface favor stimulation. When you're doing the scratching, be gentle and apply soft or moderate pressure, whichever the other person prefers.

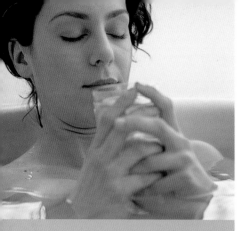

28

Choose Fresh Mineral Water

Pay attention to the source when you're choosing your water. To earn the official designation "mineral water," the water must originate from an underground source, be collected directly from where it emerged from the ground, contain a certain amount of naturally occurring minerals and other trace elements, and be free of pollution.

29 Soak in the Healing Power of Hydrotherapy

Some spa-goers believe that hydrotherapy is the closest thing they'll ever find to the fountain of youth, crediting bathing in mineral waters with the power to keep them looking and feeling young. Enjoy some of the benefits of mineral water at home by preparing a restorative bath that will not only make you feel wonderfully relaxed but will also go a long way toward enhancing your sense of general well-being.

Fill your bathtub with very warm water, enough to completely cover your shoulders. Add a handful of scented mineral bath salts to the water and mix them with your hand until they completely dissolve. Ease into the tub, lie back (use a bath pillow or rolled-up towel to cradle your neck, if you like), and close your eyes. Rest in the softening bath for at least 20 minutes, breathing slowly and deeply.

30 Hydrate Well While Bathing

Before getting into a mineral bath, pour yourself a tall glass of chilled mineral water and place it within easy reach of the tub. To make it even more refreshing, add slices of lime, lemon, or cucumber. When you're immersed in very warm water, you'll perspire, so it's important to keep your body well hydrated. Sip the cool mineral water as you soak.

After you've finished bathing and have dried yourself off, be sure to refill your water glass and keep it nearby; you'll want to continue drinking plenty of water after the treatment to stay hydrated.

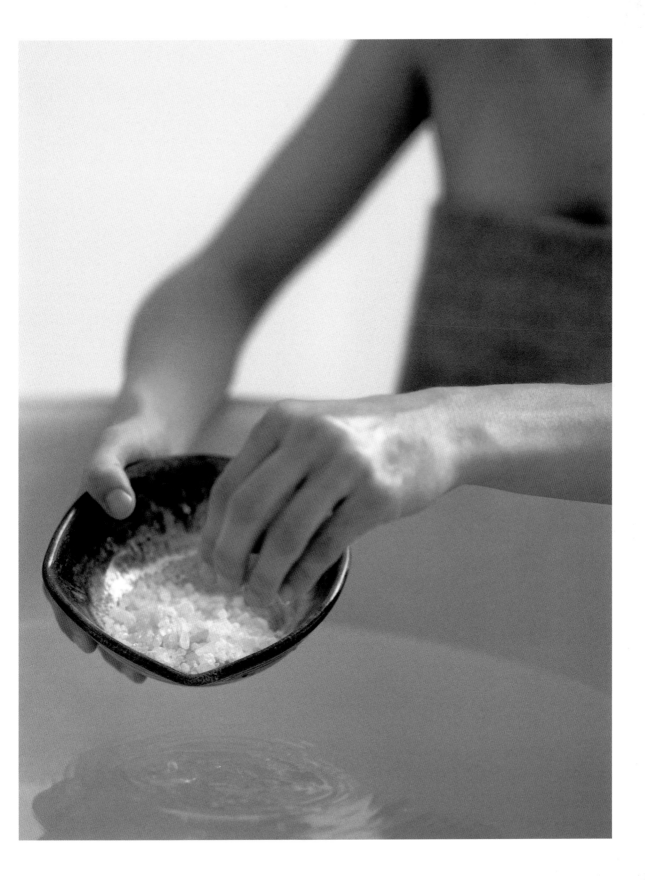

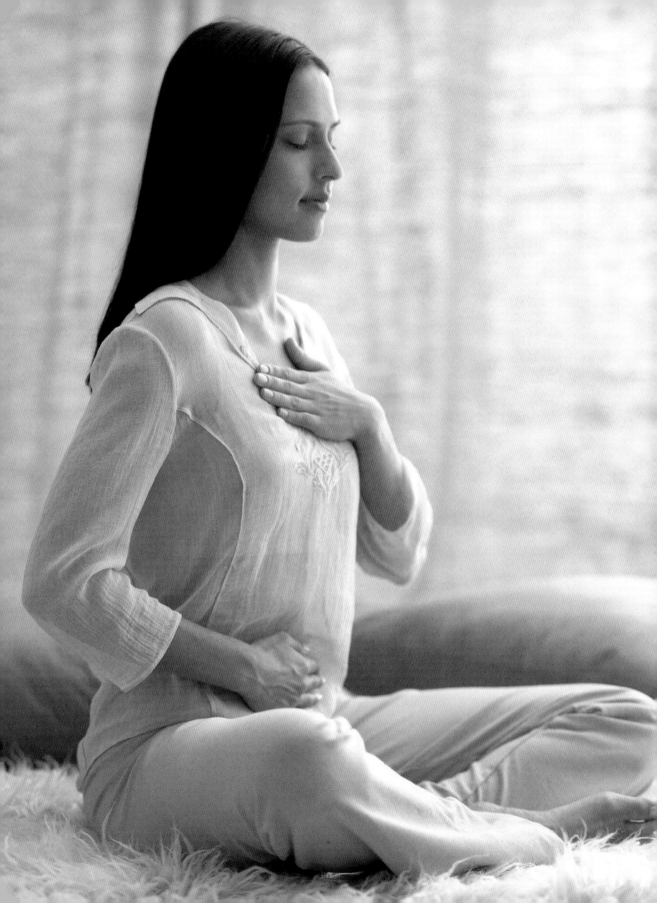

31 Practice Traditional Yogic Breaths

By bringing you into the moment and expanding the capacity of your lungs, this yoga breathing practice can provide a path to profound relaxation. Called *Deergha Swaasam* in Sanskrit, the Full Yogic Breath has long been thought to help practitioners develop concentration, clarity, and attunement with the heavens because it allows them to conjure up so much *prana*, or life force. This traditional practice also is extremely grounding and calming.

To begin the breathing exercise:

1 Sit comfortably on the floor or in a chair.

2 Inhale through your nostrils from your abdomen upward, expanding your belly and rib cage, then lifting your collarbones with the rise of your breath. Try to use the full capacity of your lungs.

3 Exhale in the opposite order, first letting the area just below the collarbones empty of breath, then your rib cage, and last your abdomen.

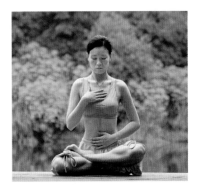

Track Your Breaths

If it's hard for you to track the course of your breath (this becomes easier with practice), put one hand on your abdomen and the other on your chest, so you can feel your body moving with your inhalations and exhalations. Just breathe slowly and deeply this way for a few minutes as you enjoy this calm, contemplative state.

32 Inhale the Benefits of Deep Breathing

"Relax and take a deep breath." Although those who proffer this common piece of advice may not realize it, the benefits are medically proven. When you inhale fully and slowly, the receptors in your lungs will signal your cardiovascular system to relax, triggering a decrease in heart rate. Deep breathing also floods your body with oxygen—its primary fuel—and opens your chest, which yogis say stimulates the heart chakra (an intersection of energy channels in the body), the spot associated with love and expansiveness. Simply breathing deeply and slowly can calm and nourish you anytime, anyplace.

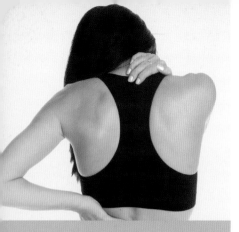

33

Precheck Pain Points

To get the most out of a massage, take the time beforehand to pinpoint spots that could use some extra attention. Do some gentle head rolls to identify tight areas in the neck, for instance, or a few shoulder shrugs and rolls to isolate troublesome areas near your shoulders.

34 Swap Neck Massages with a Friend

Recruit a friend to give you a stress-busting neck massage that will undo all those knots and kinks, and help get your mind thinking clearly again. To prepare for this relaxing massage treatment, sit backward astride a comfortable chair and rest both of your palms on the top of the chair's back. Then have your friend follow these directions:

1 Standing in front of the chair (facing your friend's back), lean your forearms on top of your friend's shoulders. Start by pressing down with one arm. Hold for three slow breaths, then release your arm. Repeat with the other arm. Then press down with both forearms at the same time as your friend inhales and lifts her shoulders, pushing them into your forearms. On an exhale, keep pressing as your friend relaxes and rolls her head in a slow circle.

2 Have your friend place her elbows on the top of the chair's back and rest her forehead in her hands. Now press the pad of one of your thumbs into the muscles at the base of her skull. You should use firm pressure, but check to make sure she isn't feeling any discomfort. Sink your thumb in on the inhale, and release on the exhale. Work point by point upward and outward along one side of her neck to about an inch behind her ear. Repeat this step on the other side.

3 With slightly cupped hands, press the pads of your fingers into the muscles on both sides of the top of the spine, near the base of her skull. Using small circular motions, travel down to the base of the neck. Repeat this technique three more times.

4 Hold her forehead with one hand. Grip the back of her neck with the thumb and fingers of your other hand. Gently rub back and forth across the neck muscles on each side of her spine, working from an inch below the earlobes down to the base of the neck. Slowly increase your pressure as you feel the muscles start to loosen. Repeat two times.

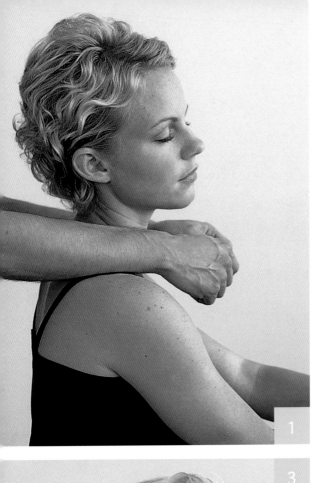

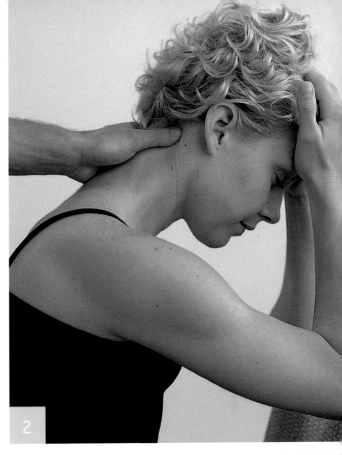

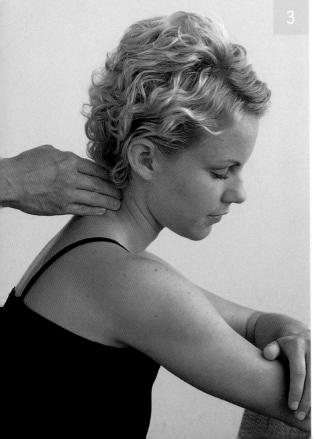

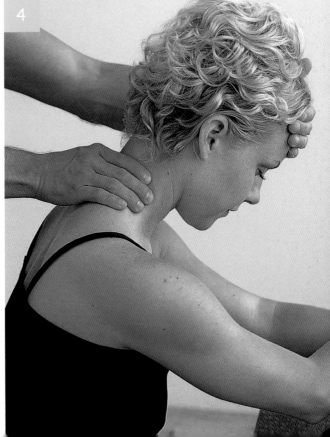

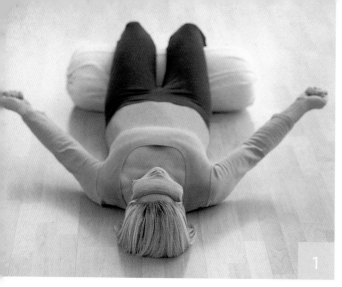
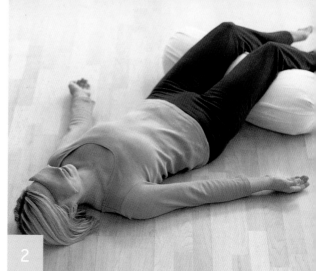

1

2

3

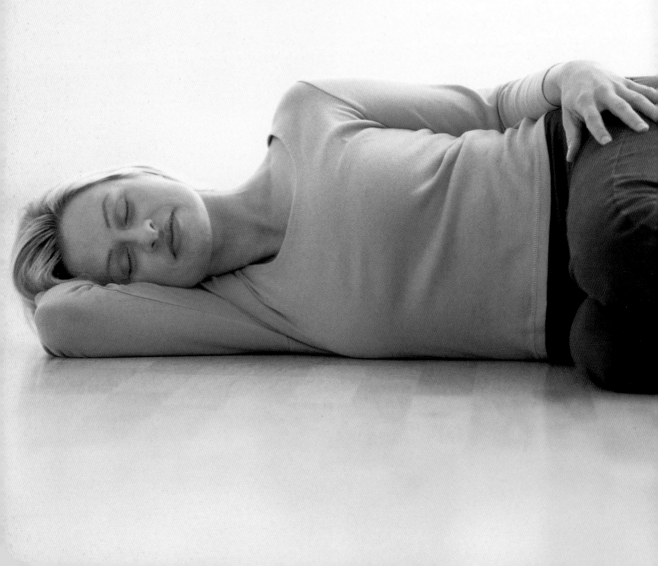

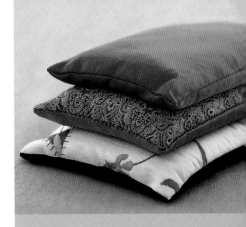

35 Sink into Deep Relaxation

Deep relaxation is a form of meditation that traditionally is performed at the end of a yoga session to allow the benefits of the poses to thoroughly permeate your body.

1 Lie on your back. Get comfortable. For additional comfort, you might want to put a pillow underneath your knees and a soothing eye pillow over your eyes. Inhale and, holding your breath, make fists as you lift your arms several inches from the floor. Squeeze your fists for a few seconds; exhale and relax, letting your arms drop to the floor. Now inhale, and then hold your breath as you lift your legs and contract your leg muscles. Exhale and let your legs drop. Next, inhale deeply to puff out your belly, and release as you exhale. Repeat with your chest. Then gently rock your head from side to side for a few seconds. Scrunch up your face; then relax it.

2 Scan your body mentally. Spend a few moments on each part as you gradually shift your focus from your toes to the top of your head. If you sense any tension as you scan, visualize that particular area relaxing and softening. You might imagine a wave of warm light slowly rising through your body, creating a perfect state of physical ease. Now take some time to observe the natural ebb and flow of your breath. After about a minute, notice the thoughts that arise in your mind, but try not to attach any feelings to them. After another minute, take the awareness even deeper, to your inner center of blissful calm. Allow yourself to fully experience this bliss for several minutes.

3 As you prepare to rouse yourself from this state of deep relaxation, spend a minute deepening your breath and enjoying the focused calm you have evoked. Then roll slowly over to your right side, cradling your right arm beneath your head; bend your knees and bring them toward your chest. When you feel ready to sit up, rise slowly. Although you are reentering the everyday world, this feeling of blissful calm will linger, leaving you refreshed and renewed.

36 Pamper Eyes with a Pillow

Use an eye pillow to add another dimension to your meditation. Made of soft fabric such as cotton or silk and filled with ingredients like buckwheat hulls and flaxseed, these pillows soothe overworked eyes by pressing upon them gently. They also block out light. Some eye pillows can be cooled or heated, while others contain calming aromatic herbs, such as chamomile or lavender.

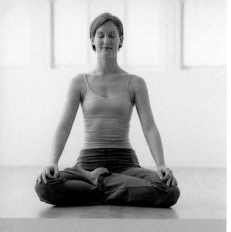

37

Sit in Half-Lotus

When sitting and meditating, beginners often just sit cross-legged. When you get more proficient, you might want to try the Half-Lotus pose. Sitting up tall, gently lift one foot and place it on the opposite thigh, sole up and close to your hip. Tuck the other foot under its opposite thigh. One leg might be more comfortable in the upper position than the other. Either way is fine.

38 Find Balance with Alternate Nostril Breathing

The ancient yoga practice of alternate nostril breathing is said to calm and balance physical and mental energies, making it especially helpful for relaxing before meditation or sleep.

1 Sit in a comfortable position, either in a chair or on the floor. Keep your back straight and your chin up. Begin to breathe deeply and regularly, and try to empty your mind of conscious thoughts.

2 When you're ready to begin alternate nostril breathing, fold the index and middle fingers of your right hand into your right palm. Close your right nostril with your thumb and exhale through your left nostril. Now inhale slowly and fully through your left nostril.

3 Now, using the same hand, close your left nostril with your ring and little fingers. Release your thumb and exhale through your right nostril. Then inhale through your right nostril and switch again.

4 Continue this pattern (exhaling and inhaling through one side and then switching to the other) for one to five minutes.

39 Stimulate Your Brain Through Breathing

Brain researchers have confirmed what yogis have long espoused: When you're breathing through your right nostril, the electrical activity in the brain's left hemisphere is stimulated, and when you breathe through your left nostril, the right hemisphere is fired up. Focus on each side as needed to reap the specific benefits.

Left hemisphere controls:
- Analytical reasoning
- Language
- Mathematical ability
- Application of order and patterns
- Focusing on details

Right hemisphere controls:
- Intuitive thought
- Creativity
- Aesthetic sensibilities
- Perception of order and patterns
- Focusing on the big picture

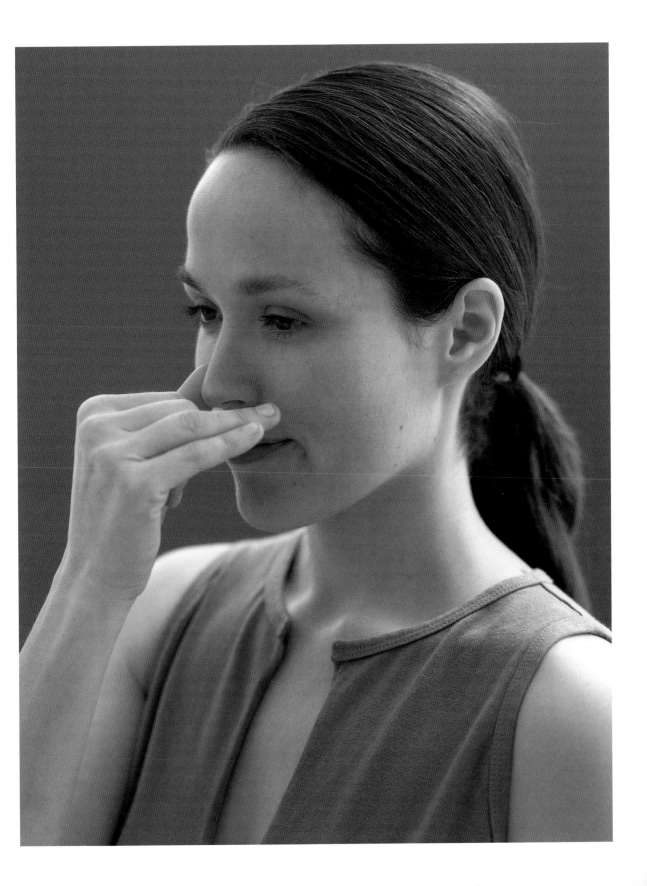

40 Unwind Before Bed with Diamond Yoga Pose

As part of your bedtime routine, try these Diamond yoga poses to calm your mind and release tension built up during the day.

1 To perform the Upward Triple Diamond pose, lie on your back in bed, bring the soles of your feet together, and let your knees sink down. Raising your arms overhead with your palms facing up, bring your thumbs and index fingers together. Let the weight of your arms and legs sink downward, bringing a sense of release to your hips and shoulders. As your body relaxes, feel your mind begin to empty. Hold this pose for one minute, paying careful attention to your breathing while keeping worries at bay, then release.

2 Now that you've begun your nighttime relaxation, move to the next phase to further your retreat from the world with the Downward Triple Diamond pose. Turn over in bed and lie face down, lifting your arms overhead and bending your elbows to create a diamond shape. Bring your thumbs and index fingers together, palms down. Bend your knees, then slide them apart and bring the soles of your feet together. Relax your hips into this pose without pressing. If you'd like a slightly more intense stretch, try gently pressing your feet downward. Hold for ten breaths, drawing your mind deeply inward. Lift your feet and bring your legs together to release.

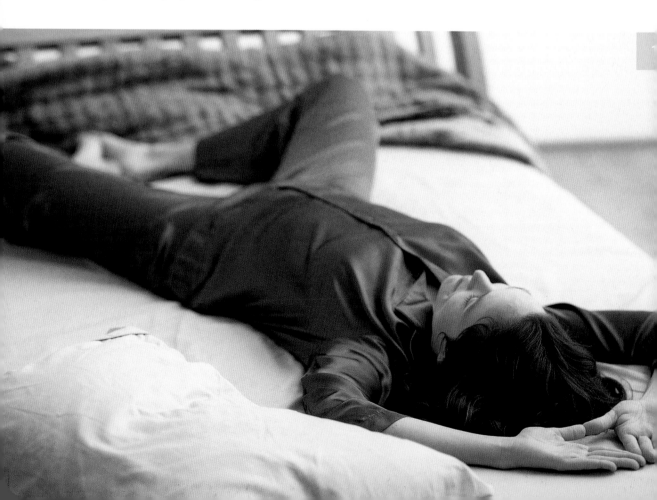

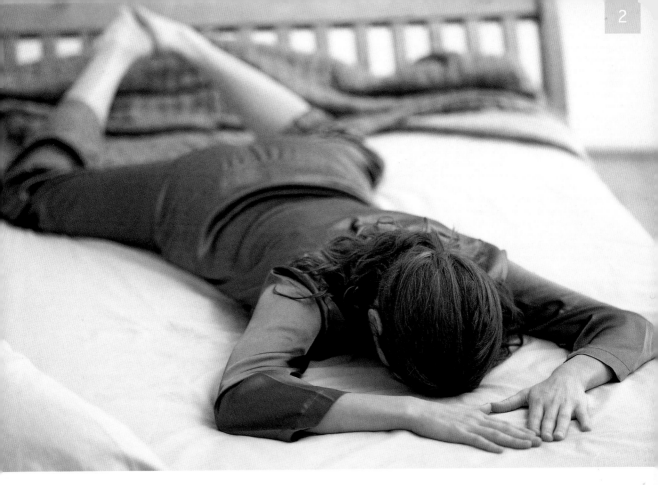

41 Fall Asleep Quickly and Stay Asleep All Night

If you often have trouble going to sleep (or staying asleep), a few lifestyle changes may help make your body and mind more receptive to a good night's rest. Perhaps the most important thing you can do is to establish a relaxing bedtime routine, such as drinking a cup of chamomile tea, listening to soothing music, reading, or meditating. Here are some other ideas for getting a little more shut-eye each evening.

- Establish a regular schedule for going to sleep and waking up.
- Don't eat heavy or spicy meals within three hours of bedtime.
- Drink alcohol in moderation, if at all, and never within two hours of going to bed.
- Promise yourself that you'll deal with worries tomorrow—just not right now.
- Make your bedroom a haven for sleep; don't do work or watch TV in bed.
- Avoid vigorous exercise within five hours of when you usually go to sleep.
- Empty your bladder before crawling into bed.
- Avoid consuming caffeine in the afternoon or evening hours.
- If you wake up and can't get back to sleep, read until you feel drowsy.

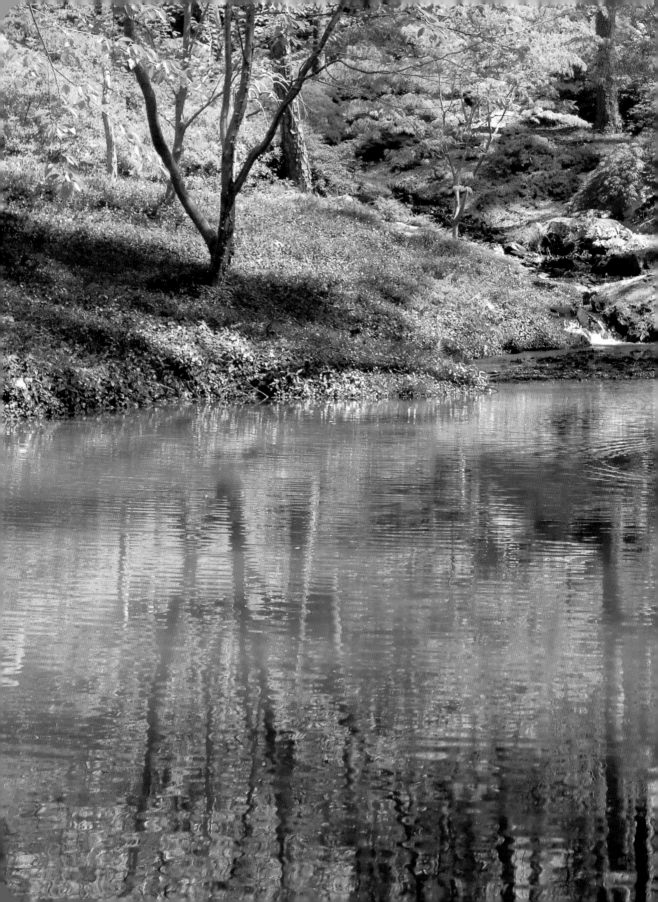

42 Practice Creative Visualization

This simple version of a classic and versatile meditation technique helps cleanse your mind by offering a welcome respite from worry. Start by finding a quiet place free from distractions, and sit in a meditative pose on the floor or in a chair with your feet on the ground, hands resting in your lap or on the arms of the chair. Relax your shoulders. Keep your spine straight and be careful not to let your chin sink down toward your chest. Now close your eyes and take a few deep breaths, inflating your lungs fully as you inhale and emptying them completely as you exhale.

After your breathing has settled into a slow, easy rhythm, begin to visualize a small pond with clear water in a picturesque setting. A bright blue sky stretches overhead, dotted with a few small, fluffy clouds that are reflected on the pond's smooth surface. Picture a pebble falling into the pond. Watch as it slowly sinks through the clear water, down, down, to the bottom. Now imagine that you are that pebble, resting lightly on the bottom of the pond, and look up toward the sky. Imagine that the clouds are your thoughts—all your worries and to-do lists. For a few minutes, just watch them drift past. You know you'll deal with them later, but, for now, your mind is still and unconcerned as you rest contentedly in your watery haven.

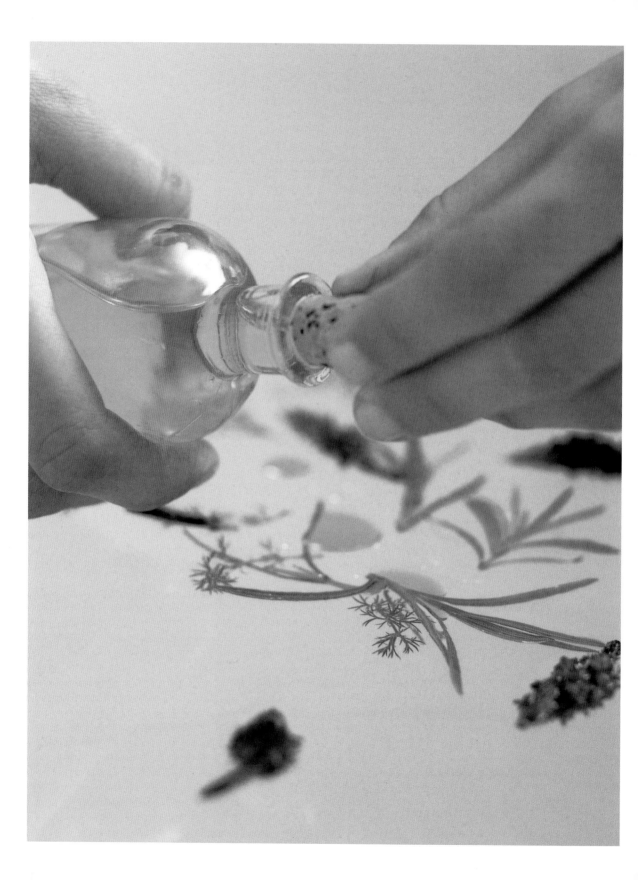

43 Dissolve Your Cares in a Lavender Bath

Lavender is probably the most popular essential oil—and with reason. A bath scented with this calming fragrance is sure to soothe both the skin and the spirit. Use lavender to dissolve away the cares of the day.

- Run a warm bath. Don't make the water too hot or you'll just end up feeling drained, not relaxed.

- Add five to seven drops of lavender essential oil blended with one ounce of carrier oil, or create a blend of lavender and other soothing essential oils (see recipe at right).

- After the bath has been filled, stir the water with your hand to evenly distribute the oil; you don't want it to pool on top, because undiluted oil might cause skin irritation.

- Lie back in the warm water, preferably using a bath pillow or a rolled-up towel under your head so you can truly unwind.

- Enjoy your bath for a half hour, if possible, topping off the bath with more warm water as needed.

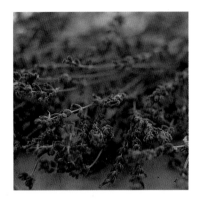

Relaxing Bath Blend

1 ounce carrier oil
7 drops lavender essential oil
5 drops chamomile essential oil
3 drops clary sage essential oil

44 Take Time Taking a Bath

When you have a chance to take a leisurely soak in the bathtub, close your eyes and let your mind empty of the chatter of the day's events. Take a mental inventory of your body, starting with the top of your head and slowly moving down, trying to identify the areas that feel tense. When you come across a tense area, contract the muscles, hold for a count of ten, and then release. Work down your body until you feel thoroughly relaxed, from head to toe.

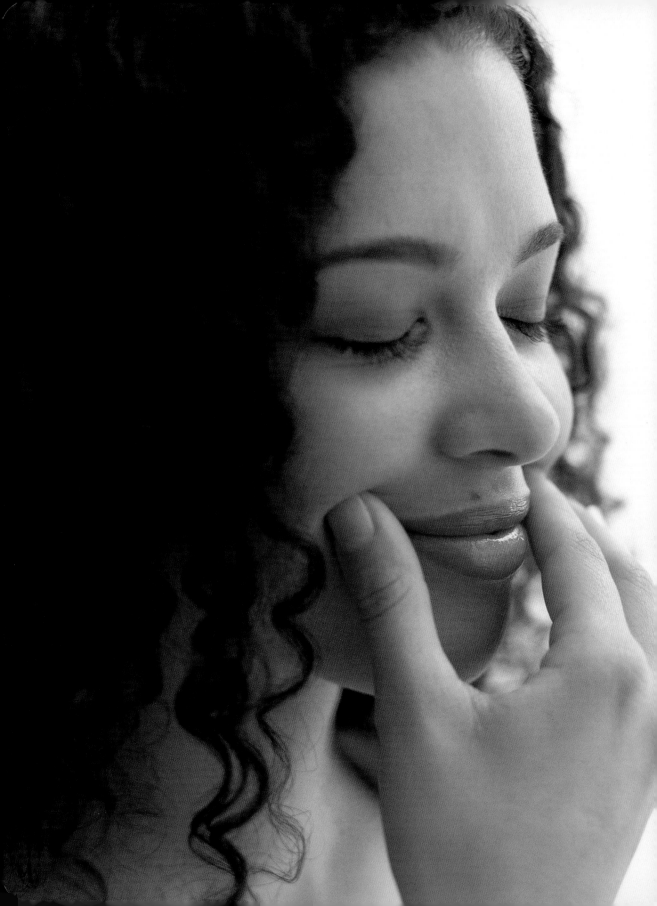

45 Cultivate your Mona Lisa Look

Consciously altering your expression can change how you feel. A simple smile can help relieve stress, depression, and self-doubt. It helps you connect with your core of happiness and reminds you not to take things too seriously. Here's a classic exercise designed to bring a smile to your face and lighten your mood.

To lift your spirits, close your eyes and smile slightly. While breathing deeply, place your thumb and index finger onto the corners of your mouth and gently push them up a little more. Feel the tension ease from your forehead. Imagine waves of joyful energy emanating from your smile and washing over your body. If there's a part of your body that you can tell is particularly tight or in distress, concentrate on sending the positive energy there. Release and repeat for ten or so smiles, until you begin to feel like da Vinci's serene lady.

Once you get used to how your body reacts when you smile in this fashion, you can achieve much of that same feeling without even changing your outward appearance (see below). This can be handy if you're sitting in a long business meeting, dealing with a difficult person, or engaged in another situation in which it might be inappropriate to break into a beaming expression.

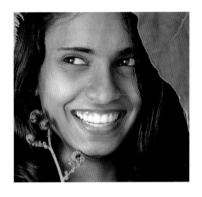

Smile to Erase Wrinkles

We primarily use five pairs of facial muscles to produce a smile, and sometimes many of the 53 muscles in our face are engaged, especially when we flash a big grin or widen our eyes in delight. (Even a slight frown takes more effort than a basic smile, and chronic frowning can create deep furrows across the forehead.)

46 Conjure Serenity on the Sly

With practice, you can learn to achieve that Mona Lisa feeling without actually smiling. Begin by creating an innocuous "physical prompt" that you can link to your Mona Lisa smile, such as putting your thumb and forefinger together. Do this physical prompt while practicing your smile; after a while, your body will actually associate contented feelings with this action. Then, when you want to lighten your spirits but it's not appropriate to break into a big grin, do your physical prompt to trigger the same warm sensations.

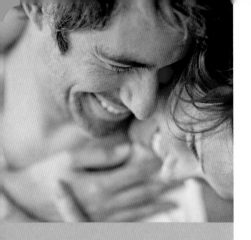

47

Connect with the Cradle Rock

To thank your partner for treating you to a massage, lie on the bed together and snuggle up behind him, resting one hand on his abdomen between his navel and ribs. Then gently rock your bodies backward and forward. This position not only feels comforting, it also stimulates the solar plexus chakra, creating a deep sense of connection between the two of you.

48 Wind Down with a Deep Massage

Sometimes you need a little help to truly unwind after a long, hectic day. Ask your partner to ease away your worries with these massage techniques before you drift off to sleep.

1 Start with a relaxing back scratch; the superficial nerves on the skin's surface love to be stimulated, even at bedtime. With your partner sitting up or lying on her stomach, gently scratch all over her back. Continue on the arms, too, if they aren't too ticklish.

2 Gentle swaying motions can be profoundly relaxing. As she lies on her back with her head in your lap, hold her hand and lift her arm to a comfortable height. For a minute or so, swing her arm from side to side, varying the speed and angle in order to encourage the release of tension. Repeat with her other arm.

3 Stroke her forehead with alternating hands for several minutes. Asian massage practitioners believe that this particular stroke helps release a buildup of excess energy in the head.

4 Finish this deep-retreat massage with a practice used by traditional healers: Put one of your hands over the other, and rest them both on her heart. Ask her to close her eyes and take ten deep, slow breaths.

49 Bond Through Touch

Massage is a powerful de-stresser: Loosening muscles, lowering blood pressure, slowing the heart rate, and decreasing the levels of the stress hormone cortisol are some of the many health benefits for the person getting the massage. But there's also a benefit for the person giving a massage beyond the satisfaction of helping another person. The skin-to-skin contact of massage floods both the masseuse or masseur and the recipient with oxytocin. Touch is one of the ways to elevate this "bonding" hormone. Oxytocin connects people emotionally, cultivates trust, and just generally makes us feel good being together.

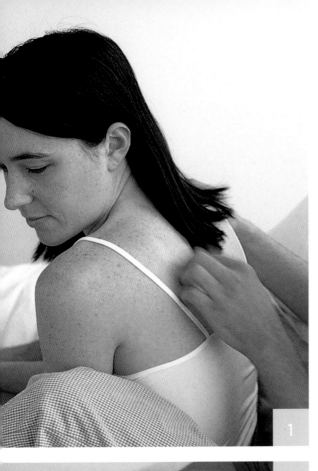

1

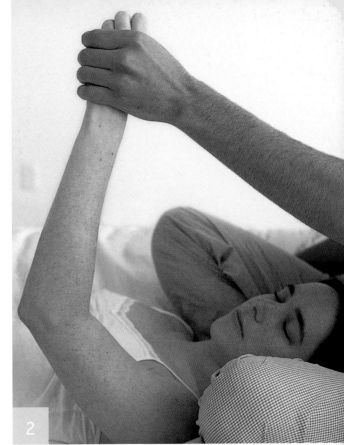

2

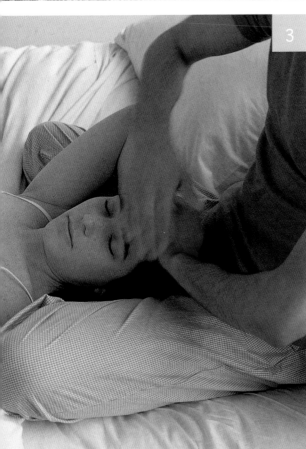

3

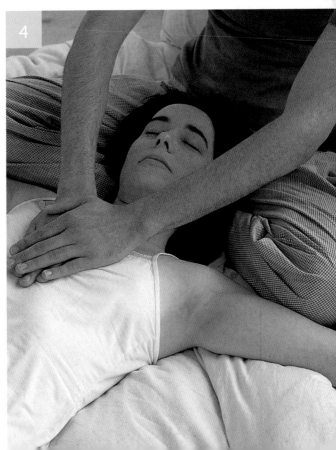

4

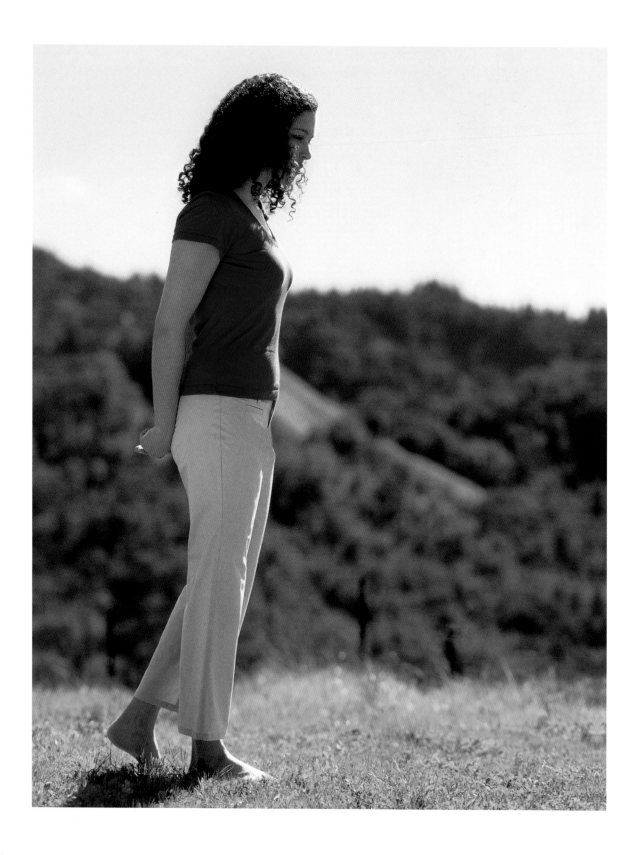

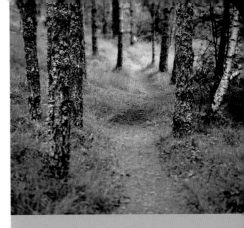

50 Free Your Mind with Walking Meditation

Practiced alone or in a group, walking can be a form of meditation. A loop path is convenient, but any path will work. Use the sensation of motion to focus your thoughts and to experience your body intensely.

1 To begin, hold your hands in any comfortable, consistent manner: loose at your sides, clasped behind your back, or in the prayer position at your heart. Be aware of your feet touching the earth and how the muscles in your body subtly work to keep you upright.

2 Start walking slowly, putting your feet down in a heel-toe, heel-toe motion. Keep your eyes open but lowered, and empty your mind of all thoughts except the sensation of moving. Feel your feet hitting the earth and then rising again. Try to keep your muscles relaxed, releasing any tension or tightness as you move along.

3 Let your mind travel up your body as you walk, registering how every part contributes to the flowing motion. If you like, synchronize each step with a breath or repetition of a mantra. (A mantra can be any uplifting word or phrase that has special significance for you.)

4 Try walking this way for about 20 to 30 minutes. When you're ready to end the meditation, just stop naturally and stand in that spot for a moment. Take a few deep breaths, notice how it feels to be still rather than moving, and feel your weight resting on the earth, all of which should contribute to your overall feeling of peacefulness.

51 Try Walking Meditation in a Group

When practicing walking meditation in a group, try having one person determine the route and set the pace, freeing the rest to concentrate on meditating in silence. Just be sure to keep two to three feet away from the people ahead of and behind you so they won't be distracted by you (and, of course, to avoid bumping into one another).

52 Meditate Anywhere

At first, walking meditation is best done on a nature path or in a place free from annoying distractions such as traffic, loud noises, and crowds (but be sure to avoid isolated areas where safety would be a concern). Once you get more experienced, you might be able to mentally block out extraneous noise so successfully that you can practice the art of walking meditation anywhere— even on busy city streets.

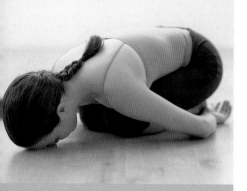

53

Stretch for Health

For the basic (not extended) Child's pose, gently kowtow, extending your hands toward your feet with palms facing up and a bend in your elbows. You can use this pose anytime to relax tension in your lower back, hips, and neck after a hard day or to unwind and rest after exercise. Breathe deeply and quiet your thoughts as you rest.

54 Ease Into Child's Pose

Curl up and retreat from the world in Child's pose. It will gently stretch your neck, back, hips, and ankles, making it a perfect resting pose when you need to take a break during yoga or other exercise.

From a kneeling position, sit back on your heels. Then lean forward and bring your chest toward your knees and your forehead toward the floor. If your forehead does not naturally come to rest on the floor, you may let your head hang or rest it on a rolled-up towel or firm pillow. Or, if you have trouble sitting on your heels, place a rolled-up towel between the back of your thighs and your calves.

To do the extended Child's pose (pictured at right), stretch your arms in front of you, shoulder-width apart and with your elbows softly bent. Reach forward with your fingertips and press down your buttocks. Gently push your palms against the floor to help you sit closer to your heels. Relax your muscles, breathe deeply, and try to quiet your thoughts for at least a minute or two. To move into the basic Child's pose (pictured at left), keep your head down and move your hands alongside your feet, palms facing up.

55 Find Spirituality in Child's Pose

The gesture at the heart of Child's pose is a bow. This symbol of humbleness and devotion is meant as a heartfelt acknowledgment of the presence of divinity and its ability to dissolve the mind's attachment to judging and criticizing others. The inward focus helps the practitioner connect with her heart, while the arms stretch forward in an offering. Body and mind rest in a position that can be seen as the embodiment of prayer. As such, this pose offers a retreat from the hustle and bustle of the external world.

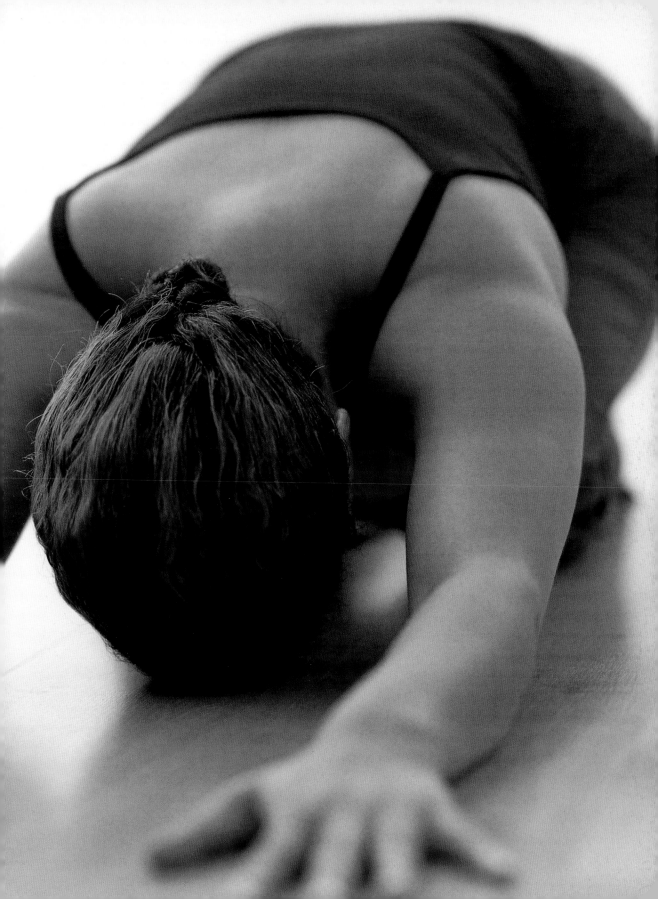

56 Enhance a Connection with Shared Breath

You share your thoughts, dreams, and embraces with your partner. Try sharing your breath with this yoga technique, which can enhance your connectedness. Sit on the floor or a bed in a comfortable position with your back resting against your partner's. The lights should be dim and the room quiet. You also can listen to soft instrumental music or a recording of nature sounds, such as a gentle rainfall.

Place your hands in a comfortable position lightly on your knees or lap and close your eyes; have your partner do the same. Focus on each other's breathing, and begin to synchronize your slow, deep breaths. If you find your mind wandering, bring it back to marking the regular pattern of your inhalations and exhalations. Practice this for as long as you both like.

As a variation, sit cross-legged and back-to-back with your partner as you inhale together and elongate your spines. Then, placing your right hand on your left knee and your left hand on the floor beside your left side (with your partner doing the same), exhale as you each turn to your own left, keeping your backs together as you twist. Hold the position for several breaths, then return to center and repeat, this time rotating to your right.

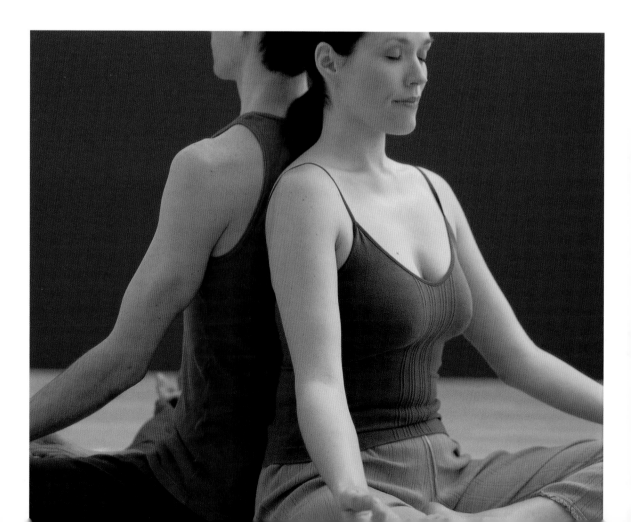

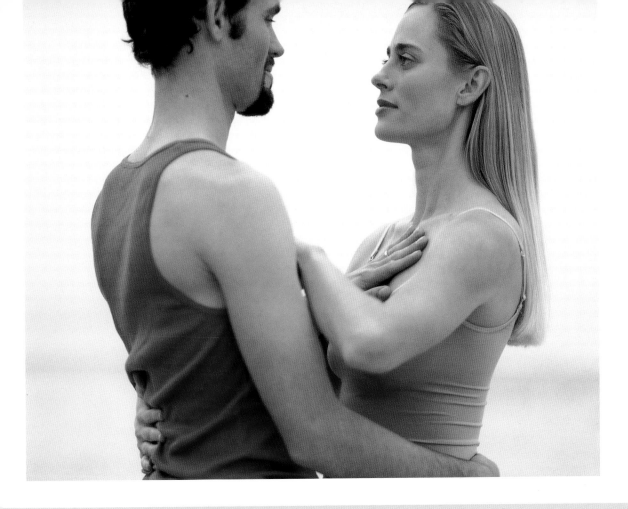

57 Feel Energy Flow with Hand-to-Heart Pose

When you share yoga practice with your partner, you develop a special awareness of each other's bodies and a state of mind that provides a quiet, peaceful way to connect. For the Hand-to-Heart pose, stand face-to-face, place your right hand over your partner's heart, and place your left hand on his or her back. Have your partner do the same for you.

Breathing slowly and deeply, gaze into each other's eyes. As you inhale, try to visualize light or energy gathering deep in your belly and rising to the crown of your head. As you exhale slowly, picture the energy cascading back down from your crown through your body. Then visualize this same effect taking place within your partner's body. Hold this pose as long as you feel comfortable and connected.

Sense the love, trust, and contentment passing between you. If one of you is troubled or hurting, visualize healing energy flowing from the other's body; if one of you has just had joyful news, feed the other with your happiness. Although this is not a physically demanding exercise, extended practice can be an intense form of meditation and intimacy.

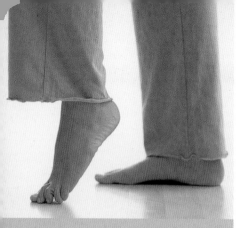

58

Use Your Toes

If you can't keep your balance on one leg (or can't do so without wobbling and hunching your shoulders or tipping forward), rest the toes of one foot gently on the ground. The key is to be relaxed and calm, not stressed by your lack of balance. That will improve with practice.

59 Get Grounded with Tai Chi

An ancient martial art that originated in China, tai chi is also known as Chinese shadowboxing. It is used as both a fighting and a healing technique, as well as a form of moving meditation. In Chinese, *tai* means "great" and *chi* means "energy," and the practice is all about experiencing, strengthening, and enhancing the flow of life energy in the body. Tai chi consists of a series of slow, graceful, and, ultimately, very powerful movements that involve the whole body and require intense mental focus. A sequence of tai chi movements is called a form, and if you practice these forms on a regular basis, they'll help you stay physically healthy, mentally sharp, and spiritually grounded.

60 Sharpen Focus with Golden Pheasant Pose

This well-known tai chi movement, sometimes called Golden Cock Stands on One Leg, helps you develop balance and stability. It also cultivates an inward focus. As you do this exercise, think of a bird showing off its plumage and picture yourself upright and elegant.

1 Start by stepping out with your right leg and placing your right foot at a 45-degree angle. Let your weight settle into your right leg. Keep your spine long and your tailbone tucked in.

2 Bend your left knee and slowly lift your left leg as high as you can while still keeping a soft angle to your knee, and point your toes down. Raise your left arm, bending the elbow up softly. Point your fingers straight up with the palm facing inward. Position your right arm down and slightly bent by your side, with your palm facing the ground. Focus on a fixed distant point to help stay balanced. Keep your shoulders relaxed and down, soften all your body angles, and maintain a straight line from the crown of your head to the bottom of your torso. Do the sequence on the other side. Then repeat on both sides once more.

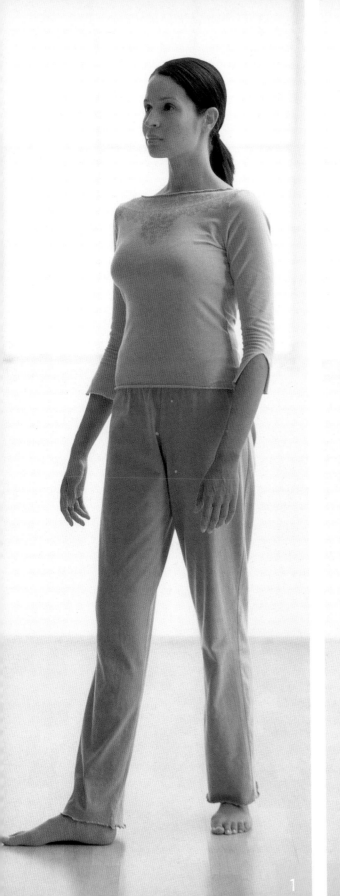
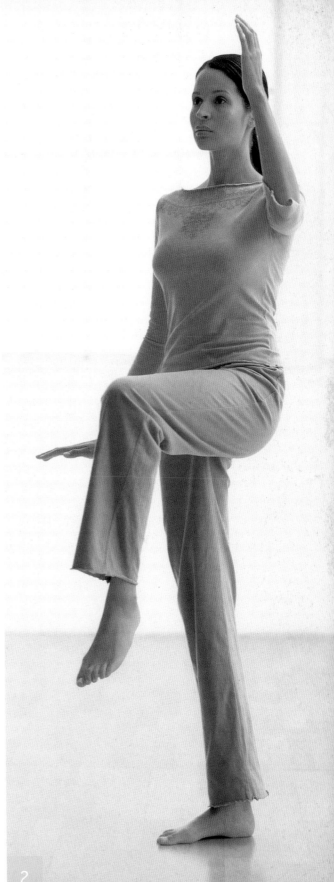

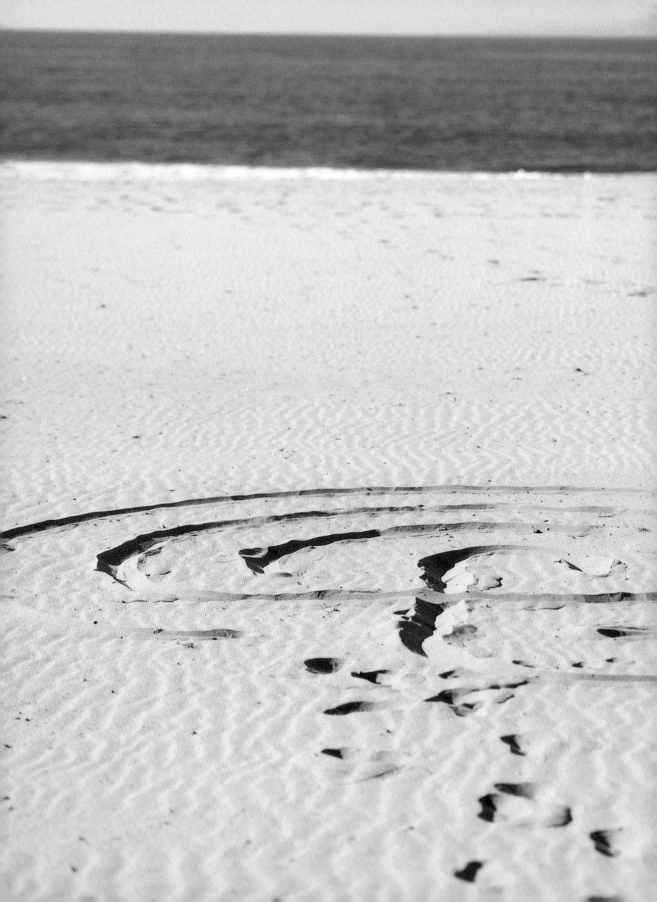

61 Walk a Path to Peacefulness

Humans have been creating labyrinths—walking paths that spiral back on themselves—for thousands of years. The ancient Greeks, Native Americans, and Mayans all used labyrinths in sacred rituals. Medieval Europeans created elaborate labyrinths for many of their churches; the French installed one of the most famous ones, fashioned of inlaid marble, at Chartres Cathedral in the 13th century. The designs and materials used may have varied greatly, but they all served as profound symbols of life, death, and mystery, a way to journey to one's own center and then out into the world again.

Today, public places such as churches, parks, medical centers, spas, and schools offer labyrinths for the public to wander. Whether you see them as symbols of life's journey, paths to salvation, metaphors for finding your own spiritual track, or intriguing vehicles for meditation, labyrinths can help you quiet your mind and find solace. If one isn't available in your area (or you're just the do-it-yourself type), you can make your own simple labyrinth in the sand or dirt.

Labyrinth aficionados bristle when one of their beloved paths is called a maze. Mazes, they point out, can have several entrances and paths, often don't lead to a center, and contain dead ends. Labyrinths have only one path; while it might twist and turn, it's simple to follow and a sojourner won't ever get lost. There are no dead ends or wrong turns. As Lauren Artress, creator of The Worldwide Labyrinth Project, explains: "A labyrinth is designed for you to find your way. A maze is designed for you to lose your way."

62 Create Your Own Labyrinth

You can make your own classical labyrinth with four easy steps. It's especially easy to draw one in sand.

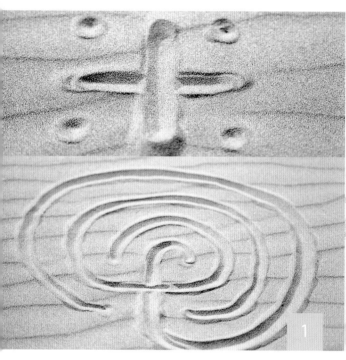

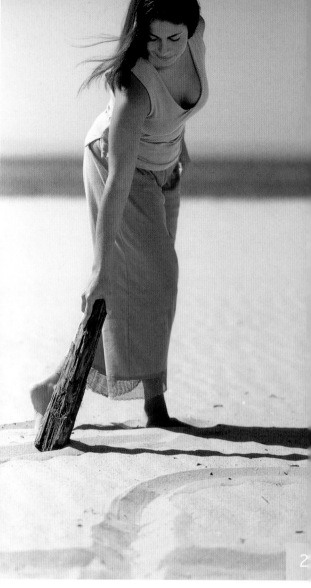

1 Draw a cross about six feet wide and place a dot in each quadrant. Next, draw four curving, clockwise lines in the following order: first, join the top of the cross to the top right dot; next, connect the top left dot to the right arm of the cross; then join the left arm of the cross to the bottom right dot; and finally, circle from the bottom left dot all the way around to the bottom arm of the cross.

2 As you draw, try to have a calm, reflective spirit. Listen to the swish of the stick as it moves through the soft sand. Feel the warm touch of the sun on your skin. Try to move and breathe with focus and deliberation. Remember that making the labyrinth can be a type of moving meditation.

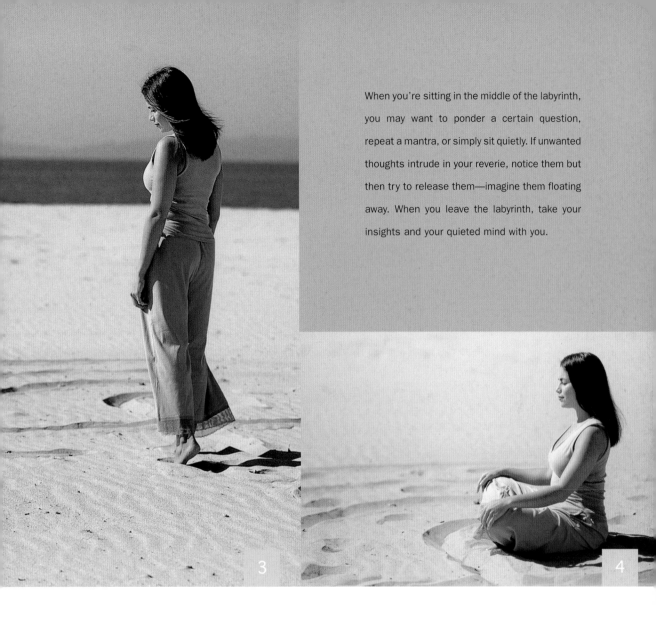

When you're sitting in the middle of the labyrinth, you may want to ponder a certain question, repeat a mantra, or simply sit quietly. If unwanted thoughts intrude in your reverie, notice them but then try to release them—imagine them floating away. When you leave the labyrinth, take your insights and your quieted mind with you.

3 When you've finished, take a deep breath at the entrance of the labyrinth and clear your mind. Acknowledge the journey you are about to begin; you may even want to formalize this by bowing, saying a little prayer, or simply closing your eyes for a moment. Choose an intention for your walk, whether it's spiritual, reflective, or playful.

4 Follow the path defined by the lines you created toward the center of the labyrinth. Try to keep your mind quiet and let go of random thoughts and worries as they arise. Concentrate on putting one foot in front of the other and breathing regularly. When you reach the center, sit and spend some time meditating. When you are ready to leave, follow the path back out of the labyrinth.

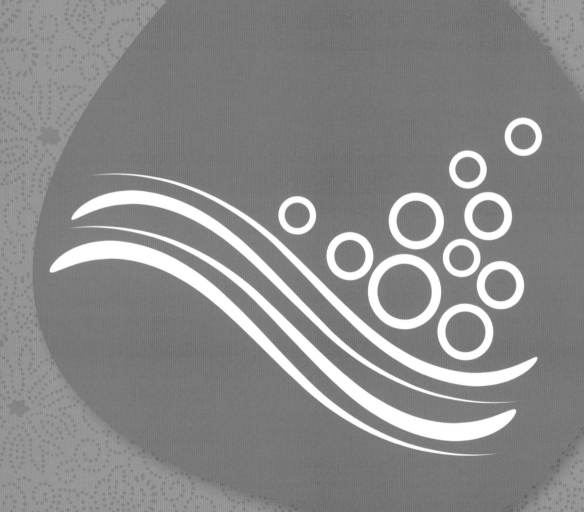

refresh

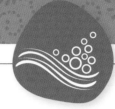

To refresh your mind and spirit, sweep away mental cobwebs and let go of negative thoughts. Keep in mind that moods are contagious, so surround yourself with positive people—or be the catalyst that changes a group's dynamics. Acting like you're happy is a simple but powerful way to make it happen.

To renew your body, create healthy habits one at a time—you might add a piece of fruit to your daily diet one week, a walk around the block after dinner the next week, and then a simple stretching routine before bedtime by the end of the month. Try one activity from this chapter at a time and stick with what works for you. These quick, easy-to-do activities are designed to cleanse and detox your body, relieve mental and physical stresses, and reveal the refreshed, healthy you in no time at all. ❧

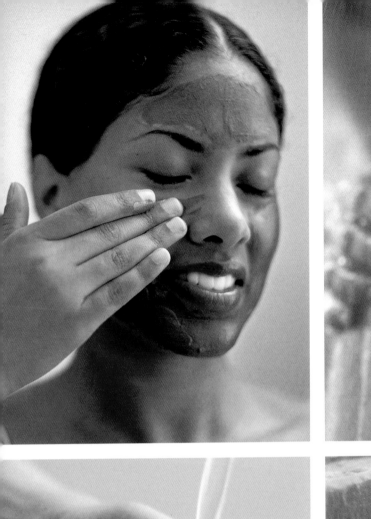
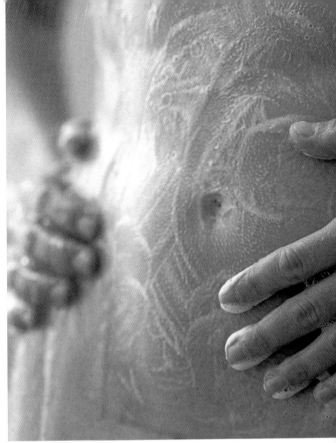
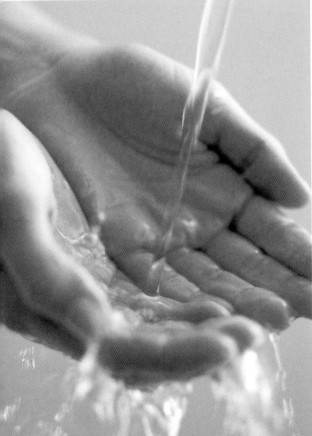
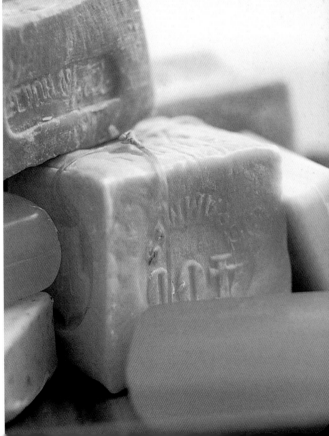

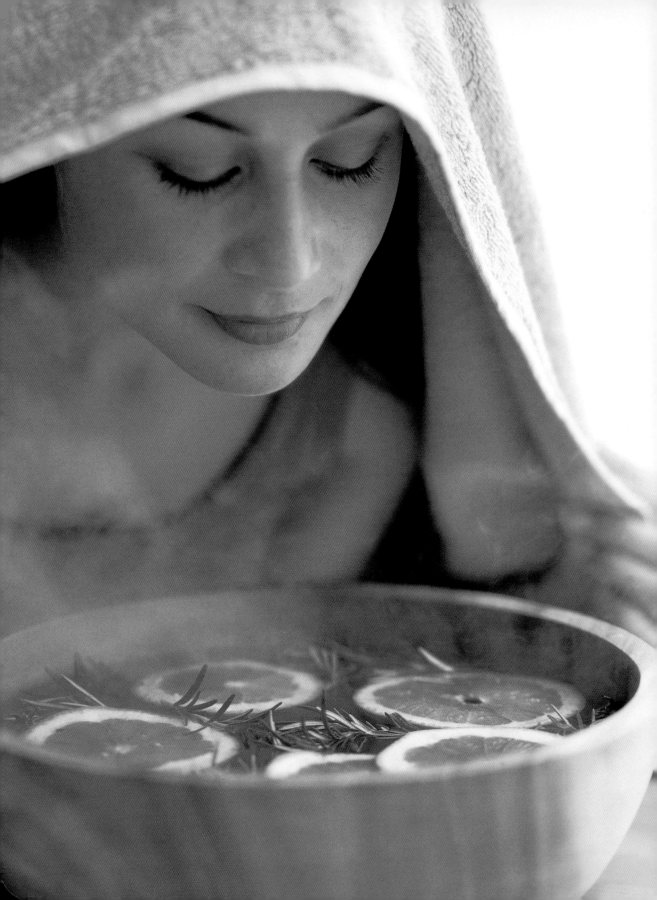

63 Add Essential Oils to a Steam Facial

Steaming opens up the skin's pores, helping to dislodge any grime and makeup residue, and imparts vital moisture to deeper skin layers. It softens dead skin cells, making it easier to exfoliate them with a gentle facial scrub. A steaming session also increases circulation to your face and relaxes facial muscles. To intensify the detoxifying effects and feel extra refreshed, add aromatic oils to the treatment.

1 Fill a bowl with boiling water. Add grapefruit and rosemary essential oils (see recipe at right), as well as sprigs of fresh rosemary and slices of grapefruit, if desired.

2 Lean over the bowl, taking care to keep your face about 12 inches away. Let comfort be your guide—steaming should be a pleasant experience, not an endurance test.

3 Drape a bath towel over your head and the bowl to trap the vapors. (If the vapors sting your eyes, keep them closed.)

4 Steam your face for five to ten minutes.

Steamed skin is fragile. Blot your face gently with a soft towel and, while your face is still slightly damp, apply a moisturizer. Top off your steam by drinking plenty of water.

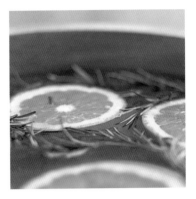

Detoxifying Steam Blend

Large bowl filled with boiling water
3 drops grapefruit essential oil
2 drops rosemary essential oil
4 sprigs fresh rosemary (optional)
4 grapefruit slices (optional)

64 Detoxify with Essential Oils

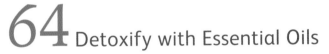

Aromatherapists often recommend grapefruit essential oil to relieve acne and tone the skin. You can use it in a steam blend or add it to a base lotion to create a healing moisturizer. Rosemary oil also serves as an astringent and an antibacterial agent that helps prevent pimples. Other detoxifying essential oils include juniper, geranium, Atlas cedar, sweet orange, and bay laurel. Experiment with individual oils and blends to find which are most pleasing and effective to you.

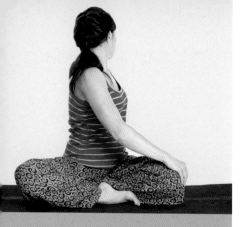

65

Twist Gently

The key to getting the most benefit out of yoga is to be gentle, to not strain, and, perhaps most vital of all, to focus on your own body's abilities. This is especially important in twisting poses.

66 Massage Your Organs with a Half Spinal Twist

While yoga poses cultivate flexibility and strength, they can also provide compression that massages the internal organs, helping to cleanse the body of toxins and provide balance.

1 Sit on the ground with both legs straight out in front of you. Bend your right knee and place your right foot on the left side of your left calf. Sit up straight and inhale as you elongate your spine.

2 Exhale as you turn toward your right, rotating from the base of your spine upward. Bring your right hand to the ground behind your back for support, and place your left arm on the right side of your leg to increase your leverage as you twist as far as you comfortably can.

3 Look over your right shoulder. Hold for 30 seconds while continuing to twist gently and breathe deeply.

4 On an exhale, untwist slowly. Turn your head forward and release from your shoulders downward as you bring your body back to center. Repeat the process on your left side.

67 Twist at Your Desk and Let Go of Tension

If you spend a lot of time sitting at work, it's important to take breaks. Try this simple twist to help release tension built up in your upper body. Sitting sideways on an armless chair with your left hip against the back, inhale and lengthen your spine. When you exhale, gently rotate to the left, working from the base of your spine upward, and grasp both sides of the chair's back. With each inhalation, elongate your spine, with each exhalation, gently increase your rotation. Visualize this twist as wringing tension from your mind as well as from your body. Hold for 30 seconds or so, continuing to take deep breaths; release gently starting from your shoulders, then repeat the twist on your other side, first repositioning your body so that your right hip is against the chair back.

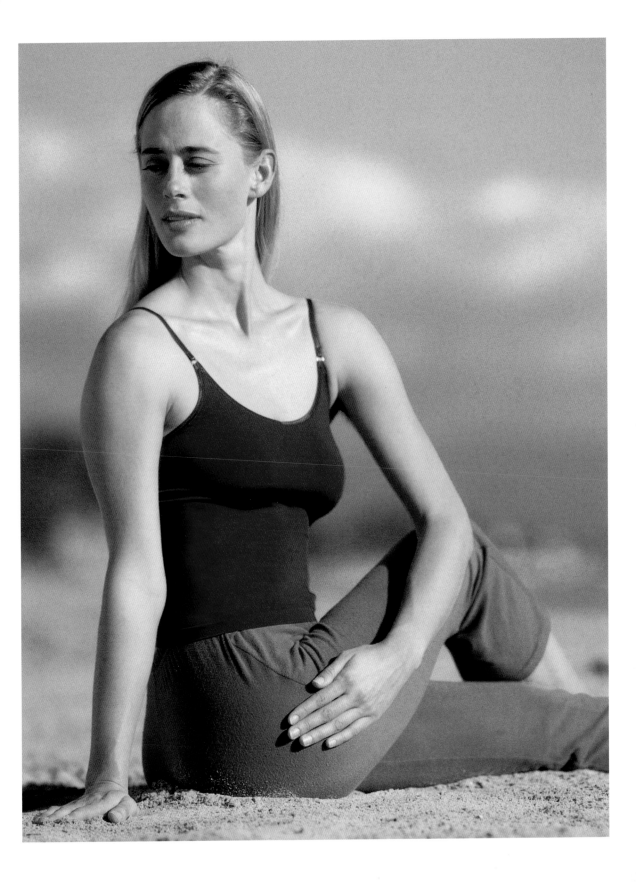

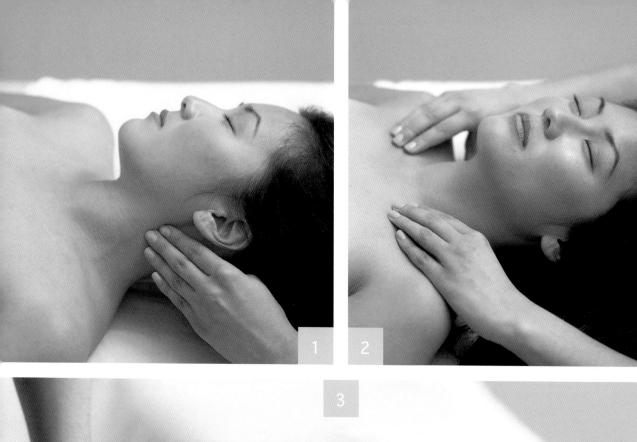

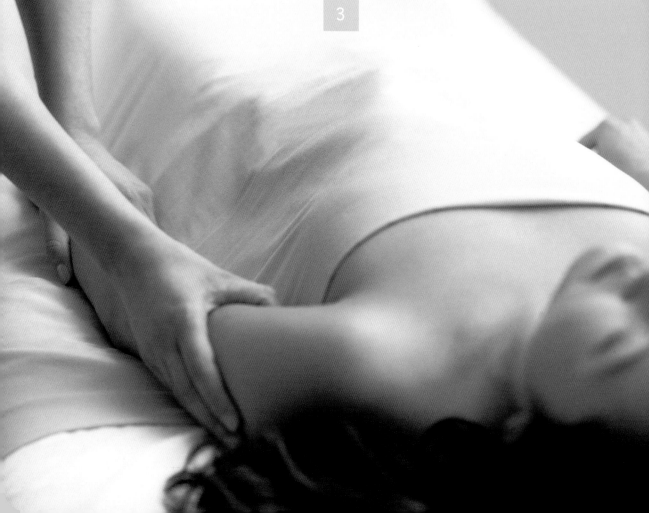

68 Glide Your Hands Deeply to Improve Circulation

Exercise, stress, and even poor diet can leave irritating chemical deposits between muscle fibers. Flushing those chemicals out helps muscles respond better and faster with less fatigue. Deep gliding massage strokes create a sweeping effect on the fluids of the body, which helps loosen these deposits. Deeper gliding also improves blood circulation, as the strokes help move blood back toward the heart and lungs to load up on oxygen for another trip through the body. Use heavier pressure when stroking toward the heart, lighter when stroking away.

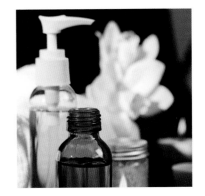

69 Get Refreshed with a Detoxifying Massage

This firm and targeted massage gives you the benefits of deep gliding strokes (see above) while lying down on your back. Ask a friend to follow these massage steps:

1 Pour a little room-temperature massage oil onto your hands (see the recipe at right if you want to use a homemade blend with essential oils). Starting an inch or so below her ear on the thick muscles at the side of her neck, use the pads of your fingers to glide lightly down the neck's sides, angling in toward the breastbone.

2 With fingers flat on top of her breastbone, sweep out across the chest muscles to the front of the shoulders. Sweep your hands back around and under her shoulder muscles and press firmly toward the base of her neck. Glide up the muscles along each side of the spine in the neck to the base of her skull. Repeat Steps 1 and 2 five times.

3 Stabilize one of her forearms with one hand, and wrap the fingers and thumb of your other hand around her forearm. Press in and glide up to the shoulder. Curve around the shoulder and glide lightly back down her arm. Do this five times and then repeat on the other arm. Move to her legs and position your hands so they overlap and wrap around one of her ankles. Then press in with your fingers and thumbs and lightly glide up to the knee. Lighten the pressure more as you move over the knee itself, then glide from knee to hip and back down to the ankle. Repeat five times, then massage the other leg.

Detoxifying Massage Blend

2 ounces carrier oil of choice
8 drops cypress essential oil
8 drops juniper essential oil
5 drops lavender essential oil
4 drops orange essential oil

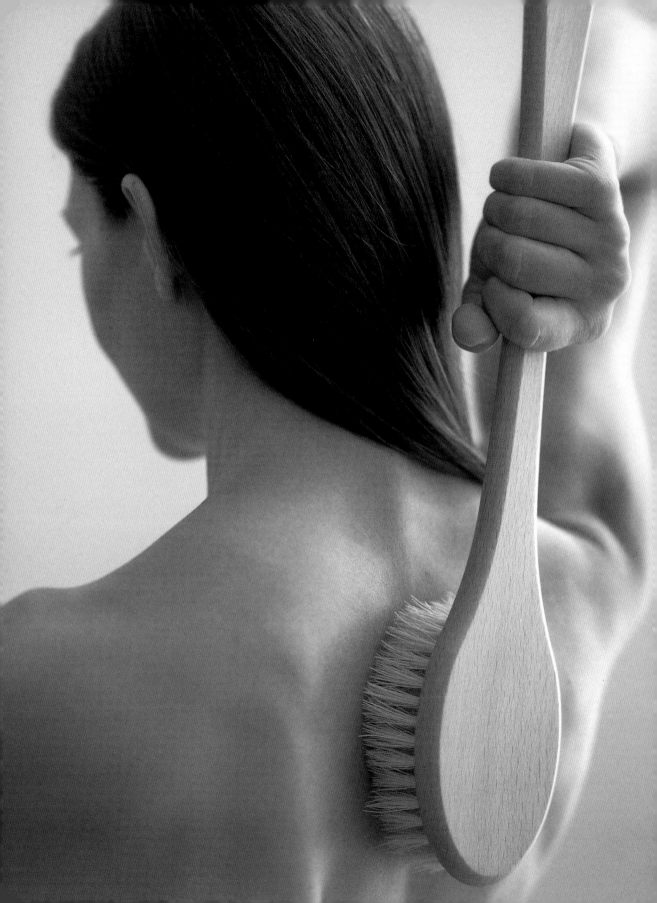

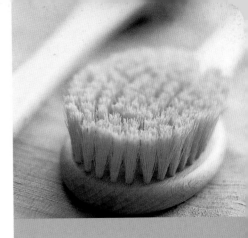

70 Rev It Up with a Brush

On those days when you feel like you need an extra boost to get up
and go, energize yourself with this simple two-step treatment designed
to rev up your circulation. Dry brushing your body before you get in
the shower helps increase circulation and exfoliates your skin as well.
Following dry brushing immediately with a shower during which you
fluctuate the temperature of the water also increases circulation, which
intensifies the stimulating effect.

1 Use a long-handled brush with soft, natural bristles and always brush
toward your heart (that is, downward when working on your shoulders
or upper back, upward when working on your limbs) Dry brush your
body starting with your back. Apply light pressure and brush where
you can comfortably reach. Then gently brush your arms, shoulders,
abdomen, legs, and buttocks.

2 In the shower, wash with soap and rinse off your body. Decrease the
temperature of the water and rinse with cold water for 15 seconds.
Adjust the temperature of the water back up to warm for a minute or
so. End your shower with a five-second blast of cold water.

71 Brush Away the Years

As we age, our skin cells refresh themselves at a slower rate, and skin
can look dull or dry, especially in winter months. Dry-brush exfoliation
removes that outer layer of cells safely, exposing the fresh, glowing skin
beneath and clearing clogged pores and other imperfections. After
exfoliating, finish by slathering on a rich, emollient moisturizer.

72

Get the Basics on Brushes

Look for a dry body brush
with bristles of natural
fibers such as cactus or
Japanese palm. Many
brushes have long handles
for hard-to-reach places.
Never use a body brush on
varicose veins, or if you
suffer from psoriasis,
eczema, or skin irritations.

73 Find Balance with Repulse Monkey

When the world gets to be too much, graceful tai chi movements can help restore a sense of balance. Take a step back with the Repulse Monkey sequence, literally and figuratively.

1 Round your arms in front of you as if holding a large ball. The right arm is down, with the palm facing up; the left arm is up, with the palm facing down. Step your left leg out. Sink down, bending your knees. Keep your tailbone tucked in and your head up, so you create a long line from the crown of your head to the bottom of your torso. Lift your left heel and point your toes down. Concentrate your weight on your back leg. Your right leg will feel "full," while your left feels "empty."

2 Step backward with your left foot. At the same time, bring your left hand around and down and your right hand around and up.

3 End with your left hand down by your belly button, palm turned up, and your right hand reaching out in front of you, at about ear level, fingers pointing to the sky, palm facing down. Your right leg is now extended in front—toes down, heel up—and feeling empty; your left leg should feel full. Repeat steps 1 through 3 on the other side (step back with your right leg, with the left arm down and the right up). Do two to four times, alternating right and left sides.

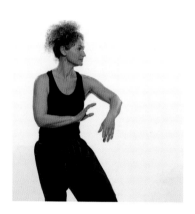

Tactical Retreats

We often think the way to win a fight is to attack. But in tai chi, the idea of yielding (or yin) is as important as thrusting forward (or yang). Tai chi emphasizes the ability to adapt and respond to an opponent's actions, and sometimes retreating is more powerful than resisting, attacking, or otherwise trying to win—and that's the case whether you're in a verbal argument or involved in hand-to-hand combat.

74 Move and Meditate

For Westerners accustomed to a bombardment of external stimuli, it isn't always easy to quiet the mind and gain full awareness of the body. Yet even for folks who are easily distracted during sitting meditation, tai chi can provide a form of moving meditation that's more engaging and effective. The emphasis on slow, controlled movements, inward focus, and proper body alignment compels the practitioner to concentrate and be fully present in the moment.

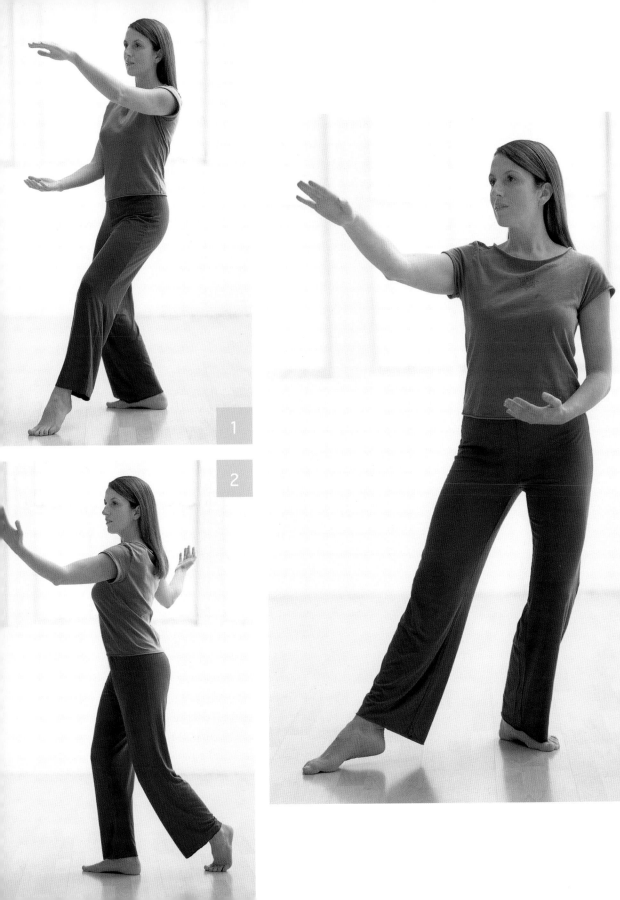

1

2

3

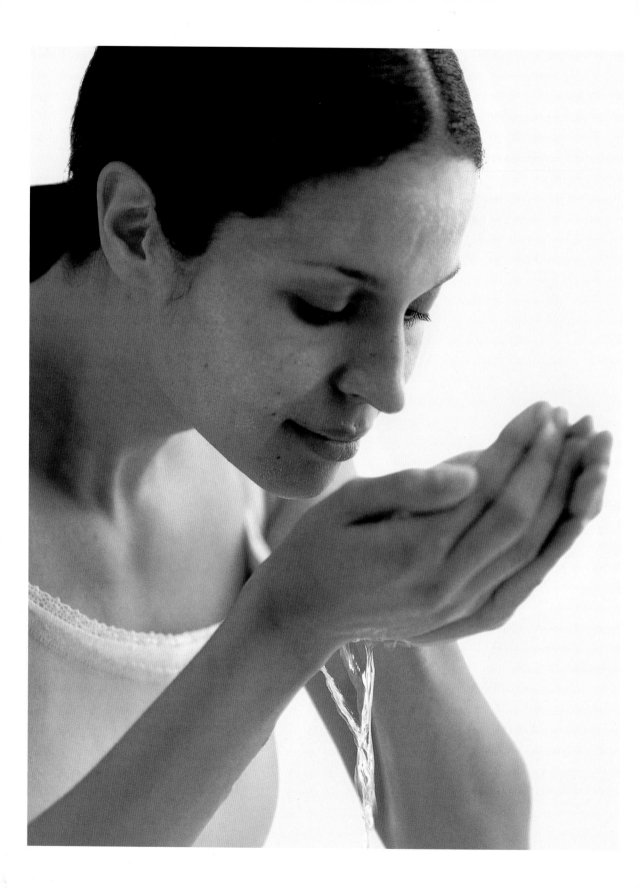

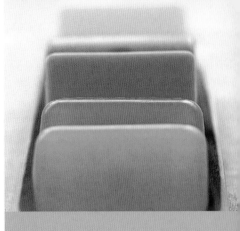

75 Deep-Clean Your Face

We all wash our faces but, admit it, sometimes not so thoroughly—or we skip cleansing altogether before we hit the hay for some shut-eye. Washing your face well, though, is an important step to keeping facial skin looking and feeling its best. Wash your face in the morning and at night unless you have dry skin (if so, you can skip the morning).

Start by washing your hands thoroughly (see below), then wash your face for at least 30 seconds, using a cleanser formulated for your skin type. Dry skin frequently benefits from a cleansing milk or cream. Normal skin can tolerate many forms of cleansing products, and which type you settle on is a matter of personal preference. (If you use a foam or bar-soap cleanser and your skin feels tight and dry shortly after washing, try switching to a slightly more emollient product.) Oily skin usually responds well to a refreshing foam or gel. If you have combination skin, you may need to cater to the oilier areas of your face, and then take care to moisturize the drier areas.

76 Wash Your Hands Well

Washing your hands often is one of the most effective things you can do to stay healthy. The catch is that the cleaning needs to be thorough enough to prevent illness from spreading.

Despite the multitude of antibacterial soaps and hand sanitizers on the market, you just need soap and water, according to the Centers for Disease Control and Prevention. Once your hands are wet and soapy, rub them together to make a lather. This is the critical part: scrub them well, including the backs of your hands, between your fingers, and under your nails. Continue rubbing your hands for at least 20 seconds (it's longer than you think: set a timer the first couple of times to get a feel for it). Rinse your hands well under running water. Dry your hands using a clean towel or air dry.

77
Choose Your Soap

Soaps break the rule that oil and water don't mix. A component of soap called surfactant has a molecular structure that attracts water on one end and non-water-soluble substances on the other. When you lather up, surfactant links oil (and dirt) to water; simply rinse and off come the dirt and oil adhered to it. If you find that a soap is too harsh for your skin, it may have too much surfactant. Try a milder option.

78 Exfoliate All Over to Reveal Radiant Skin

Manual exfoliation helps the body shed dead skin cells, exposing healthier-looking, more radiant skin waiting just beneath. As you shower or bathe, spread a small amount of cleansing gel on a sisal washcloth or mitt, or on a loofah for more intense exfoliation. If your skin is dry or sensitive, use a soft washcloth or your hands. (Never exfoliate sunburned or broken skin). Work the gel into a lather and then rub the cloth or loofah all over your body, scrubbing toward your heart to aid the flow of lymphatic fluids.

Alternatively, skip the rough applicator and use an exfoliating scrub designed for your skin type. First, cleanse and rinse off as usual in the shower. Then turn off the shower. Using a preformulated sea salt, nut, or sugar scrub (or the recipe at right), scoop out about two tablespoons into your hand and apply the scrub firmly over your skin in small circular motions, starting with your feet and legs, then your arms. Pay special attention to any patches of dry skin, such as those often found on heels and elbows. Next, exfoliate your buttocks, stomach, back, and chest, decreasing pressure when working on delicate areas and adding more product as needed. Rinse with plenty of warm water, dry off, and slather on moisturizer.

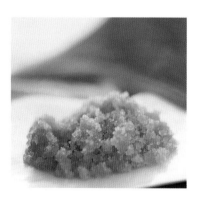

Sweet Body Scrub

2 tablespoons granulated sugar
1 tablespoon brown sugar
4 tablespoons honey
2 teaspoons lemon or lime juice

79 Expose a Whole New You

The body sheds up to 500 million dead cells daily from the skin's upper layer, the epidermis. If these cells remained, they would form a thick layer, locking out moisture and making the skin appear dull or flaky. Exfoliating helps the body slough off dead cells, revealing a new layer of rosier skin. It also helps stimulate circulation, loosen ingrown hairs, and lift away dirt and excess oil. As we age, dead cells take longer to rise to the top of the epidermis and then slough off, so exfoliation becomes an increasingly important self-care ritual.

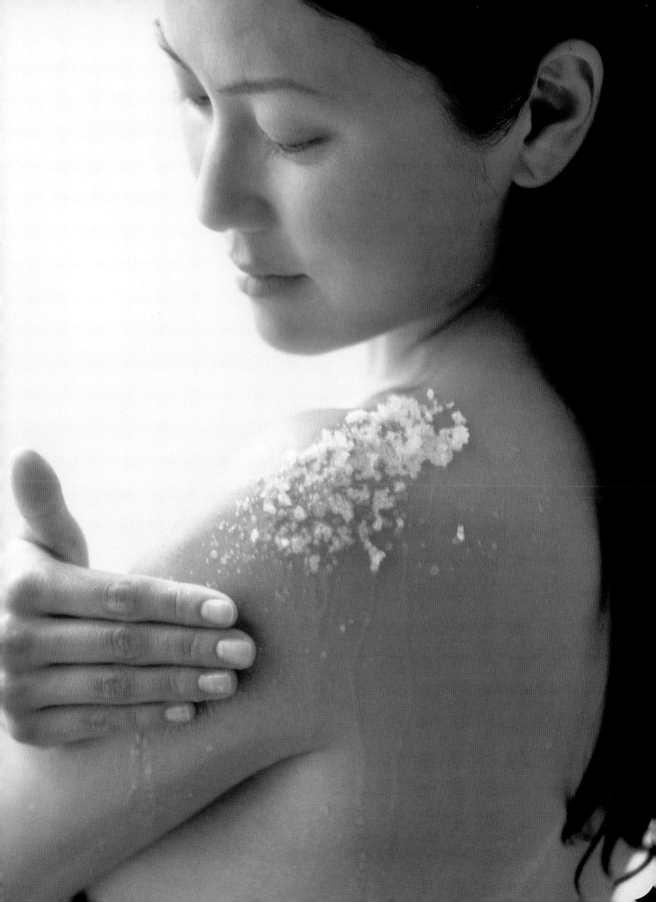

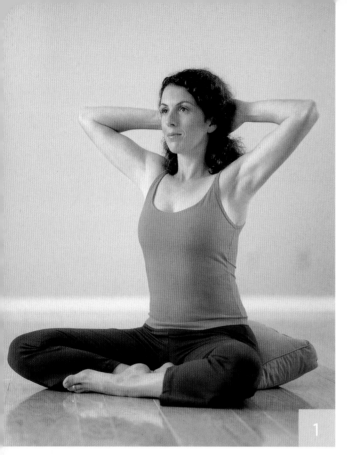

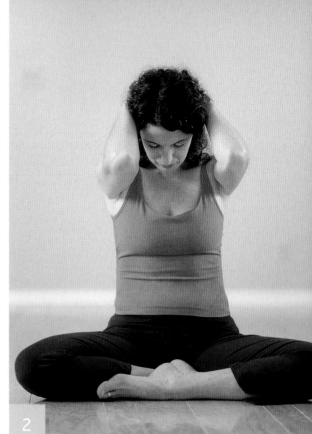

1

2

3

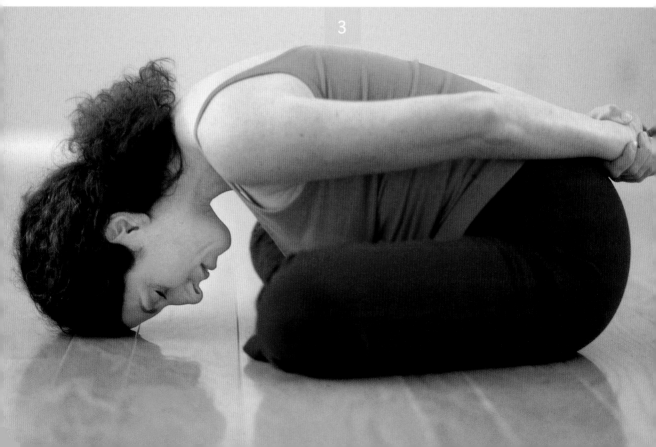

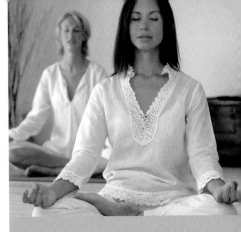

80 Get Centered by Releasing Spinal Tension

Feel calm, centered, and ready to go after performing these two yoga poses, which release tension in your neck, shoulder, and back muscles.

1 For Folding Wings pose, sit comfortably cross-legged on the floor, elongate your spine, interlace your fingers, and bring your hands to the back of your head. Inhaling, press your elbows back, press gently on your head, and open your shoulder blades wide.

2 Exhaling, fold your arms alongside your ears, lengthen the back of your neck, and bring your chin toward your chest. Then inhale as you lift your head and press your elbows back again. Repeat these opening and closing movements for four breaths.

3 Add to this feeling of relase by doing Yogic Seal pose. Staying in the cross-legged position, bring your hands behind your back, and gently grasp the wrist of your dominant hand with your other hand. Inhale and elongate your spine, then exhale as you fold forward from your hips. Keep your hands relaxed against your back. Let your head hang toward or rest against the floor. If this is uncomfortable, place a firm cushion, a folded blanket, or a rolled towel under your head. Direct your mind to a place of utter stillness. Hold for 30 to 60 seconds, then slowly sit up on an inhalation.

81 Arch into a Stretch

From a comfortable seated position, place your right hand on the floor at your right. Lift your left hand up with your thumb facing back. Inhale and stretch upward, than exhale and arch to the right. Let your right arm bend, reach your left arm to the right, and look forward. Keep your chest up and hold the pose for four to eight breaths, inhaling as you straighten up. Repeat on the other side.

82 Breathe Well

Try to pay careful attention to your breathing when you practice yoga. In yoga, inhalation usually is linked to movements that expand the chest and abdomen, and exhalation is keyed to movements that compress the abdomen. When you hold poses, try to breathe through your nose, and never hold your breath, which can strain your body, unless specifically instructed to do so.

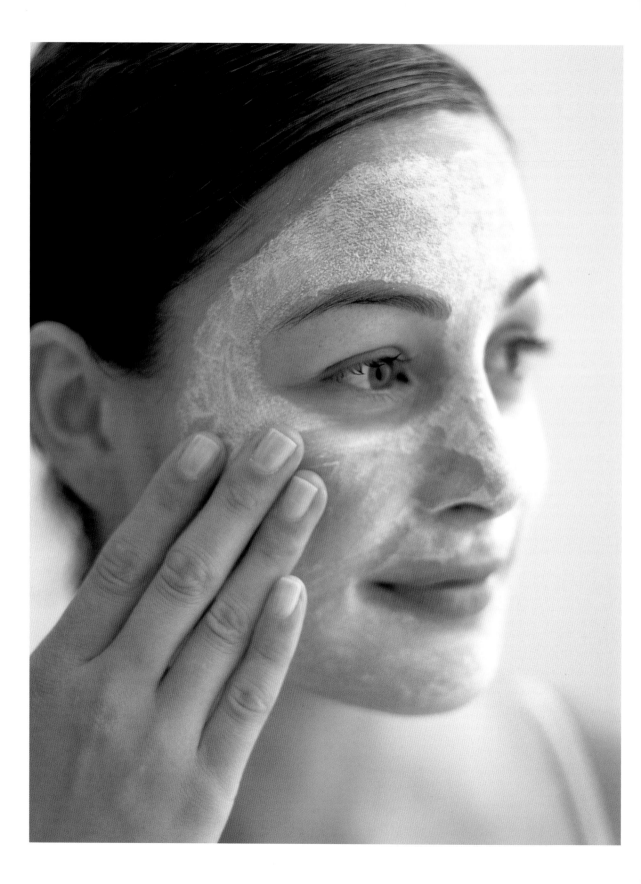

83 Tame Inflamed Skin with Tea Tree Oil

If you have oily or acne-prone skin, regular use of a deep-cleaning mask made with tea tree oil helps to minimize breakouts and keep excess shine and oiliness under control.

Oily skin is caused by overzealous sebaceous (oil) glands—or simply an overabundance of them. The greasy film that results can clog pores, encouraging pimples and blackheads, especially in the face's T-zone (forehead, nose, and chin). Tea tree oil's deep-cleaning properties help combat these problems, and its antibacterial qualities soothe blemishes and prevent new ones from forming. (Tea tree oil also can help prevent infections in cuts.)

After washing your face, apply a tea tree oil–based facial mask (many excellent commercial products are available, or see the recipe at right for a homemade version). Spread a thin, even layer over your face, avoiding the lip and eye areas. Leave it on for ten minutes. Remove the mask by rinsing your face with warm water and wiping away any residue with a moistened washcloth.

A tea tree oil–based moisturizing gel softens and hydrates your skin without being too heavy or irritating. Apply about a quarter-sized squeeze of gel onto clean fingers and massage it into your skin.

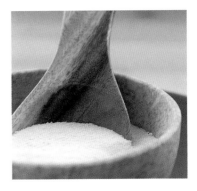

Deep-Cleaning Mask

1½ tablespoons kaolin (white clay, pictured above)
1 tablespoon oat flour
3 to 4 tablespoons orange juice
1 tablespoon finely chopped mint leaves
1 teaspoon extra-virgin olive oil
5 to 8 drops tea tree oil

84 Moisturize Every Skin Type

Even oily skin needs daily moisturizing. Some recommendations from the American Academy of Dermatology: Use a moisturizer that is lightweight and noncomedogenic (does not block pores) and contains a broad-spectrum sunscreen with an SPF of least 30. Avoid products with cocoa butter, cinnamon, and coconut oil. A mild retinoid at night followed by a moisturizer to stimulate collagen production can help prevent fine lines and wrinkles and reduce irritation. Be careful not to over-wash oily skin, which can cause it to dry out. When your skin gets dried out, your body increases oil production, resulting in more frequent breakouts.

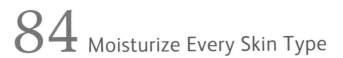

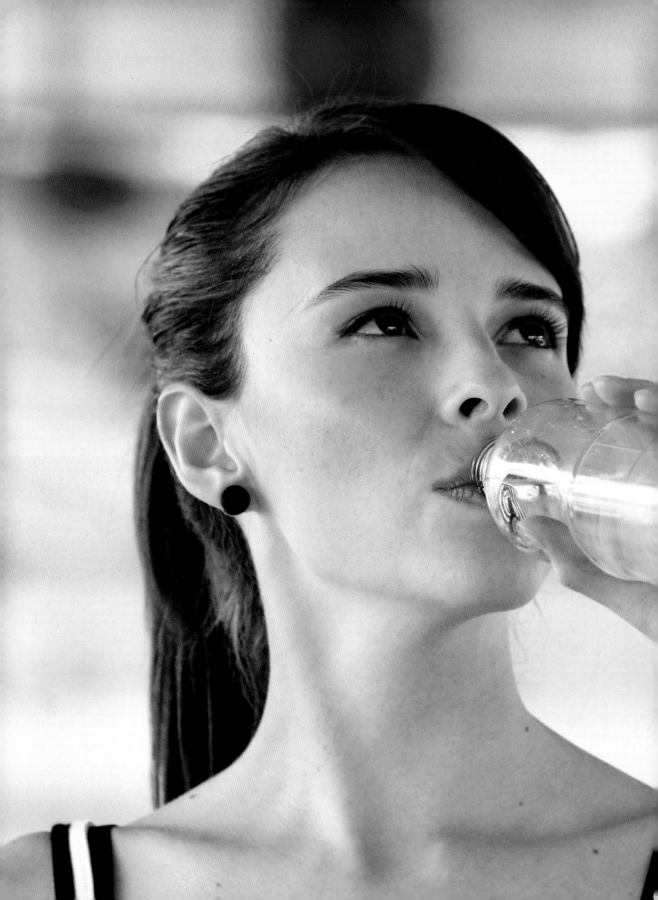

85 Hydrate for Health

You can find lots of exotic potions on the market touting all sorts of health benefits. But one of the simplest (and least expensive!) is water. After oxygen, your body needs water more than any other substance. Every system in the body depends on water to function correctly. Water makes your skin supple, lubricates joints and muscles, fights fatigue, and helps flush toxins from your body. Even minor dehydration has been linked to tiredness, memory lapses, faulty concentration, and irritability; severe dehydration can be life threatening.

So how much of this magic elixir do you really need? Everyone has heard the advice "Drink eight 8-ounce glasses of water a day." But individual needs vary, and physical activity, exposure to heat, and illness can affect your day-to-day requirements. Most healthy people drink enough by consuming beverages at meals and when thirsty. The Institute of Medicine recommends that women consume approximately 91 ounces (2.7 liters) of water each day. In addition to plain water, you also get credit for the water in beverages such as juice, milk, coffee, and tea, as well as the water content in food, which accounts for about 20 percent of our water intake.

An easy test to see if you need to drink more: Look at the color of your urine. It should be pale yellow, roughly the color of lemonade, if you're adequately hydrated. If it's darker or strong smelling, increase your fluid intake. (Note: Vitamins and certain foods can affect the color of urine.)

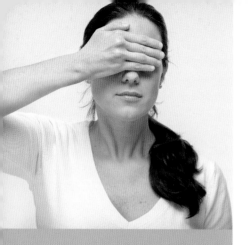

86

Enhance Relaxation

To supplement the relaxing effect of the forehead sweeps, release built-up energy around the head by doing a few broad strokes as well. Close your eyes, and cover your forehead with one hand, resting your palm and fingers across your brow. Lightly stroke up from your eyebrows to the top of your head. Switch hands and repeat. Alternating hands, do about two dozen strokes.

87 Massage Your Forehead

A forehead massage aids lymphatic drainage and shifts facial muscles from habitual positions. Not only does facial massage relieve tension, it actually can enhance your appearance. Massaging improves blood circulation, which helps impart a radiant glow, and it also relaxes the tensed muscles that can give a weary, pinched look to your face.

1 Relax in any comfortable position. Close your eyes, and place the middle finger of each hand on the innermost corners of your eyebrows (the part nearest your nose).

2 Applying gentle but firm pressure, slowly trace a path from just above your eyebrows to your temples. (Firm pressure helps ease muscle tension.) Return to the starting position.

3 Sweep out again, this time moving just below your eyebrows to your temples. Take care to press on the brow bone, not your eyes.

4 For the third pass, trace a path from the innermost corners of your eyebrows up to your hairline. Glide your fingers across your forehead and down to your temples. Complete three sets of sweeps.

88 Keep Skin Smooth and Youthful

The movement of facial muscles creases the skin, and aging—with its attendant loss of collagen, facial fat, and oil production—can turn those creases into furrows. Add the sun's effects and smoking (researchers have found that smoking turns on a gene that destroys collagen), and you get a recipe for wrinkles. To help slow down their formation, use sunscreen and moisturizers with antioxidants, don't smoke, and wear sunglasses and a hat with a wide brim when you're outside. Massage also helps ease tense facial muscles, which helps reduce creasing.

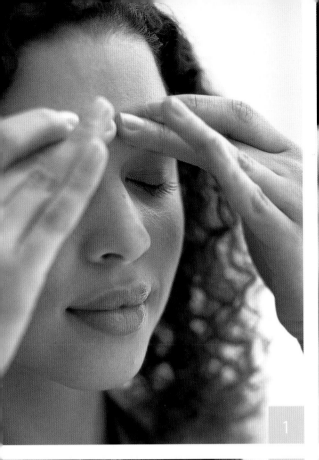

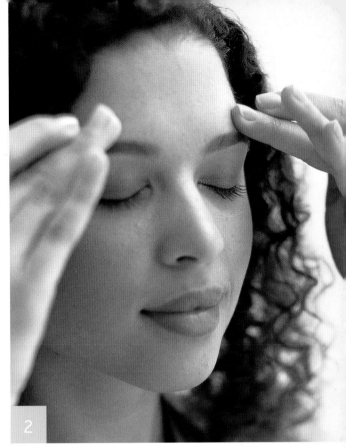

1

2

3

4

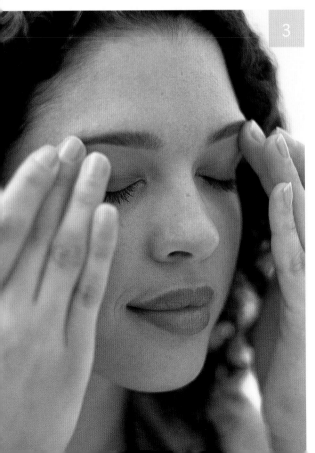

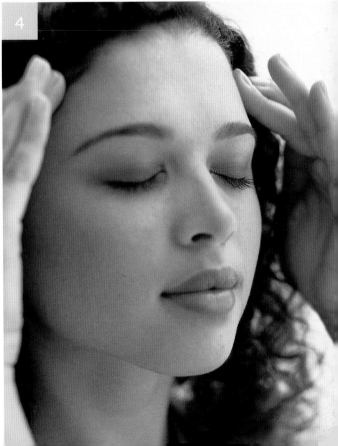

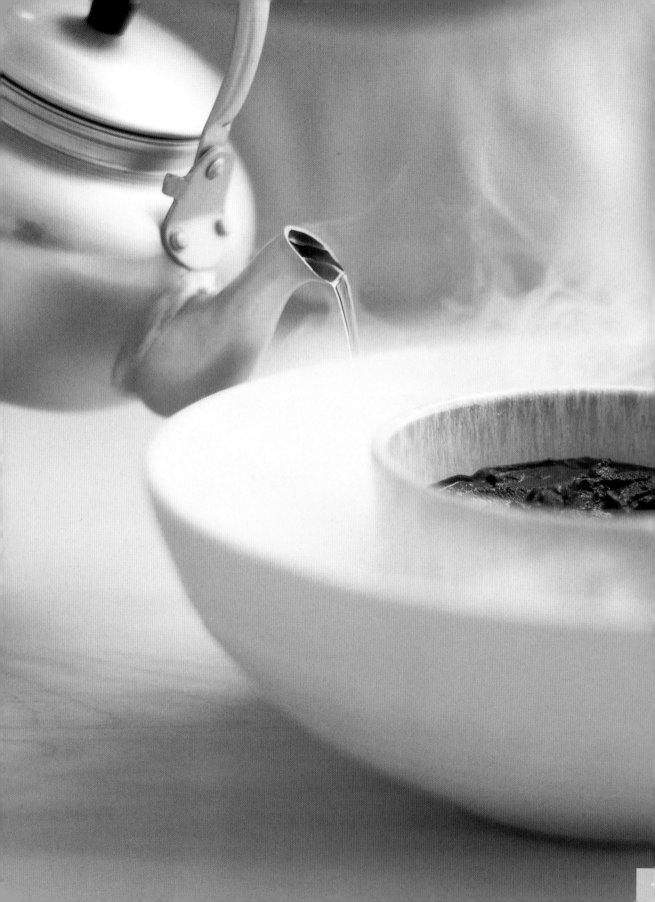

89 Make a Mini Mud Bath

When a full-body mud bath isn't a practical option, using a small amount in a spot pack is a convenient, effective way to reap some of mud's natural healing and detoxifying benefits.

1 To make a mud pack, use a thick, therapeutic body mud (it should not be runny). Scoop about one cup of the mud into a small heat-conductive bowl. Fill a larger bowl two-thirds full with boiling water. Place the bowl of mud into the bowl of water, being careful not to let the water overflow into the mud. Stir the mud occasionally.

2 Cut a piece of highly porous cloth (such as cheesecloth or heavy gauze) into a 12-by-12-inch square. Lay it unfolded on a heat-resistant surface. When the mud has heated thoroughly, take the smaller bowl out of the hot water. With a spatula, scoop all the mud out of the bowl onto the center of the cloth. Mound the mud so that it's about an inch or two thick in the center. Fold each corner of the cloth on top of the mud to form a neat pack.

3 Position the mud pack directly on any area of your body causing you discomfort. Be sure to keep the folded layers of cloth on top, and the thin, porous layer against your skin. Wind some plastic wrap around the affected area to retain the heat, then cover it with a towel. Leave the pack on for 20 to 30 minutes.

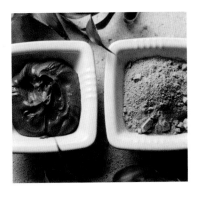

Mud Pack

1 cup thick, therapeutic body mud
1 small heat-conductive bowl
1 large bowl
Boiling water
1 12-by-12-inch square of
   highly porous cloth
Spatula
Plastic wrap
Towel

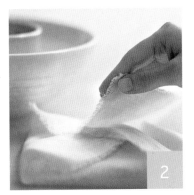

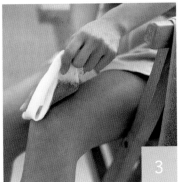

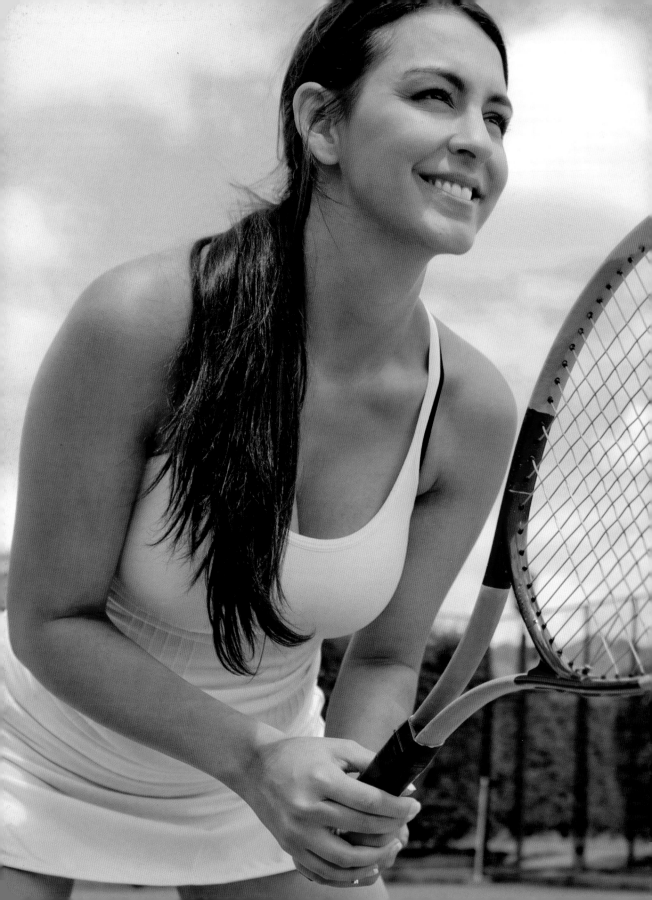

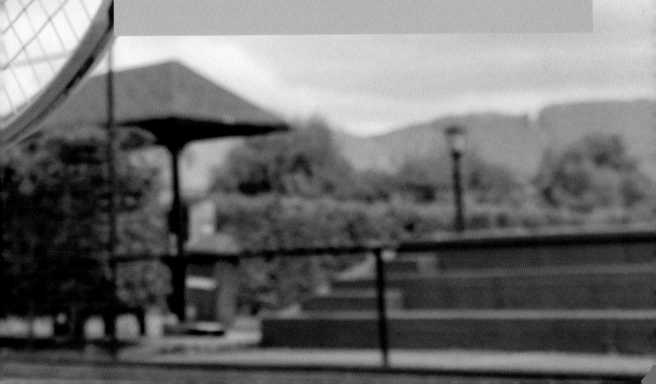

90 Work Up a Sweat

People all over the world have been using sweat to cleanse their bodies—and even purify their souls—for centuries. The Finnish have their hutlike saunas. The Russians enjoy cavernous public baths known as *banya*. Japanese *sento* offer a variety of bathing options (including hot and cold pools). Native Americans build sweat lodges heated with hot rocks to rid their bodies and minds of impurities, and to commune with the spirits.

Sweat—a mixture of water, sodium chloride, potassium salts, urea, and lactic acid—cools the body via evaporation. Whether sweat actually flushes out environmental toxins is up for debate, but getting hot enough to make your body sweat is certainly healthy. It improves blood circulation, helps rid the body of normal waste products, loosens muscles, and gives you rosy cheeks. Equally important, a good sweating session makes you feel better: cleaner, more relaxed, and profoundly renewed.

You may not have a sauna or steam bath at your disposal, but that doesn't mean you need to forgo the pleasures of perspiration. Vigorous exercise—whether it's a kickboxing class, a long run, or chasing your kids around a playground—can also help you work up a good sweat.

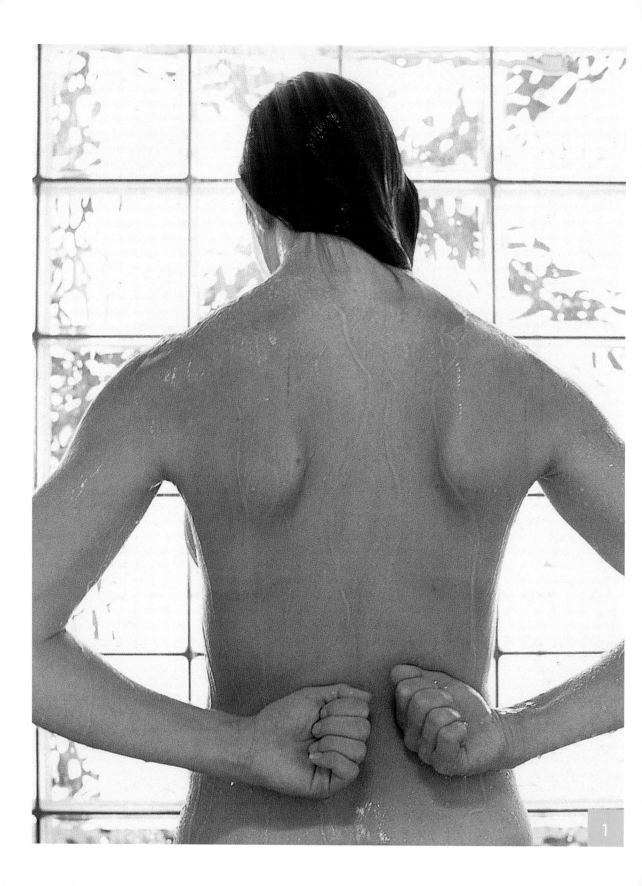

91 Detox Your System

When you've had a bit too much the night before, only time will completely clear your head and settle your stomach. But some simple detox techniques speed the process along.

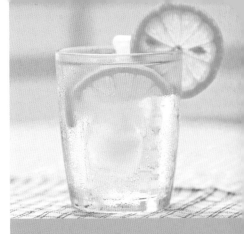

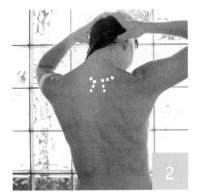 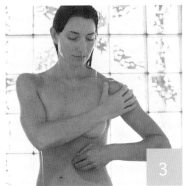

1 Lend your detoxification filters a hand by gently pummeling your kidneys. Leaning over slightly, reach behind you and, with soft fists, gently pound below your lower ribs, about 12 times on each side, using comfortable pressure.

2 To help relieve nausea and headaches, press your thumbs into the muscles and acupressure points along your skull and neck. Start by placing your thumbs at the base of your skull, one on each side of the upper spine. Press in for two breaths, release, and move an inch outward; repeat until you're an inch or so away from your ears. Return to the upper spine and press on each side again, this time inching your thumbs downward along the length of your neck until you reach the tops of your shoulders.

3 In shiatsu, the point known as Spleen 16 is a classic target for relief from hangover symptoms. Using the fingertips of one hand, find the bottom of your rib cage and move your hand directly in line with your nipple. Feel for a slight indentation in the bone, and then press gently upward into the ribs. Hold the point for a count of ten full breaths. Repeat on the other side.

92

Battle a Hangover

- Drink plenty of water to rehydrate your body; adding a little lemon juice will give the detoxification effect a boost.

- Resuscitate yourself with a cool compress on which you've sprinkled three drops of lavender, peppermint, or rosemary essential oil. If you're nauseated, use rose or sandalwood oil instead.

- Take a vitamin B supplement—granted, this is something that would be more effective if taken right before your binge, but it will still help you feel better the next morning.

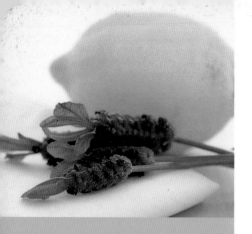

93

Alleviate Airborne Anxiety

If the thought of getting on a plane makes your heart race, try this easy technique to take the edge off your fears: Put a couple of cotton pads sprinkled with a few drops of lavender and lemon essential oils in a small resealable plastic bag, and carry it on board with you. If you start to feel anxious, open the bag and inhale the comforting scent released by the aromatic oils. Close your eyes, concentrate on breathing slowly and deeply, and meditate for a few minutes.

94 Stay Flexible in Flight

Sitting for long periods can cause muscles to stiffen and impede blood circulation. Head off problems with these stretches, which you can do discreetly in your airplane seat. During long flights (or car or bus rides), try to perform all of these steps every two hours or so.

1 To encourage deeper breathing and perk up sluggish circulation, press both elbows firmly back into your seat, arch your chest forward, and inhale and exhale three times while maintaining the pressure with your arms. Relax, rounding your back slightly. Repeat three to five times, until you feel your heart pumping a little.

2 Raise both arms over your head, bend your elbows, and grasp your left elbow with your right hand. Take a deep breath, then exhale and gently pull your left elbow to the right. Lean a little to the right and try to extend the stretch down to your waist. Hold for about two seconds, then sit up straight, rest your arms on top of your head as you inhale deeply, and repeat the stretch as you exhale, going a few inches farther each time. Then stretch your right side.

3 Improve the circulation in your legs by using the sports-massage technique of compression. Rest one ankle on top of the opposite thigh. Firmly press the heel of your hand into your calf with rhythmic, pumping strokes, working the muscles from ankle to knee. Then increase the blood flow to your legs by pointing your toes down and then up. Flex each foot this way about a dozen times.

4 Hold your right forearm with your left hand. Place the top of your right fist just above your right knee. Press down on your right leg with the flat of your knuckles; bend your body forward for added strength. Release, move your fist an inch or so toward your hip, and repeat. Cover your entire thigh this way, rhythmically rocking your weight forward and back. Then switch sides and repeat on your other leg.

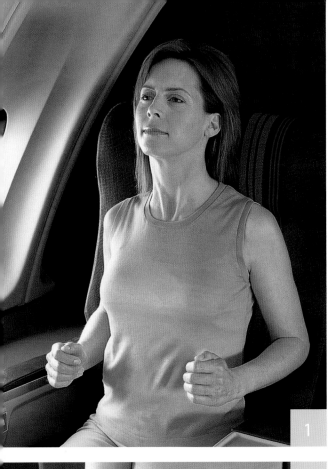

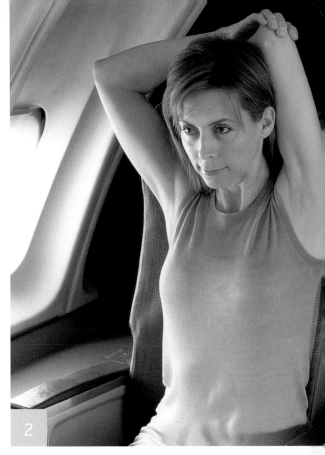

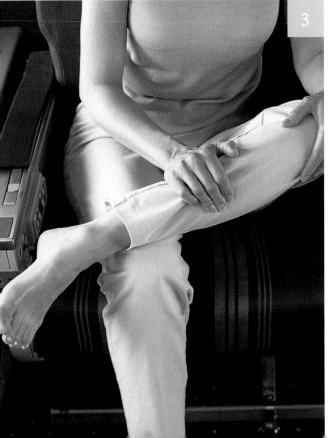

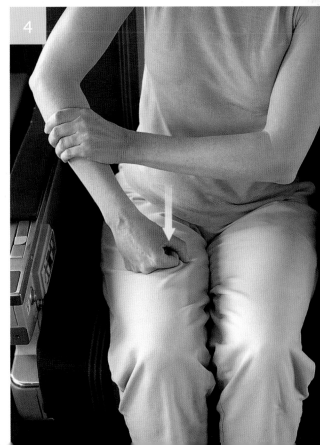

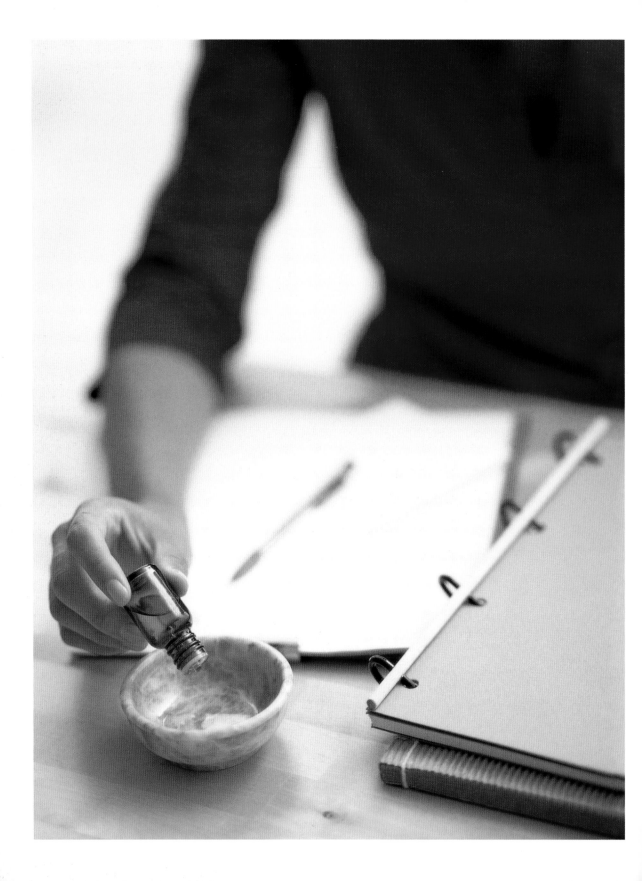

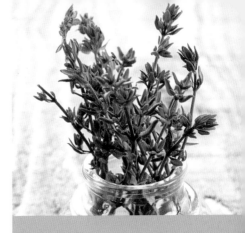

95 Keep Your Office Healthy

Most workplaces are, by their very nature, bad for our health. All those colleagues, customers, and clients sneezing and coughing, all that stale air circulating and recirculating. You may not be able to fling open your windows or persuade your coworkers to stay home when they're under the weather, but you can enlist a powerful ally in the fight against office germs: essential oils. A good number of them have been shown to possess antibacterial, antifungal, and antiviral properties. The aromas of most of these oils also have beneficial psychological effects and, in some cases, are said to help boost the immune system.

Germ-killing essential oils include thyme, tea tree, spike lavender, pine, fir, rosemary, and eucalyptus. Diffusing these scents throughout your office is an excellent way to activate their therapeutic qualities. Electric diffusers are best for this purpose because there's little risk of overheating the oils, thus destroying some of their potency, and they circulate the scent efficiently. You also can add a few drops of your chosen essential oil to a little water in a small bowl and place it in your work space, or drizzle a few drops onto cotton balls and put them near (but not on) a radiator or heating vent.

One good-neighbor caveat: Keep in mind that the fragrance you find delightful might seem downright offensive to your office mates. Ask your coworkers if they mind any of the oils you use, and try to pick a few that everyone finds appealing (or at least inoffensive).

96 Energize in an Instant

Rather than relying on caffeine, eliminate tiredness and raise concentration levels at work with essential oils: peppermint, to refresh and stimulate; lemon, to uplift and enliven; and sweet orange, to balance and lift moods. Use any of these oils with a diffuser, or sprinkle a little oil on a tissue and keep it at your desk. (Avoid direct skin contact when using undiluted essential oils.)

97 Supercharge with Thyme

With its antiseptic, antibacterial, antiviral, and antifungal properties, thyme (pictured above) is one of the most potent germ-killers in the aromatherapist's arsenal. Be careful, though: While appropriate for use in a diffuser, the type of thyme essential oil that contains carvacrol (a strong antiseptic) is too harsh for skin contact.

98 Boost Immunity with a Torso Twist

By stimulating the lymphatic and endocrine systems, and quieting the central nervous system, yoga can help keep you healthy and fit. For this immune-boosting pose, stand with your feet together and your arms hanging loosely by your sides. Begin to twist your torso gently from side to side, allowing your arms to swing and bump lightly against your body. Gradually increase your speed so that the force of your swings lifts your arms away from your body. Continue for a minute or two to stimulate the lymph glands in your underarms.

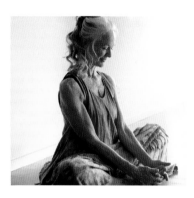

Revive Your Immune System with Yoga

Because of its meditative, calming nature, yoga induces a state of relaxation. When the body is relaxed, it releases fewer stress hormones, which have a negative impact on the immune system. Relaxation also encourages the body to produce endorphins, which boost the immune system, reduce pain, and activate the brain's so-called pleasure centers.

99 Relax in a Right Angle

Lie on your back facing an unobstructed wall. Your back should be perpendicular to the wall, and your knees should be slightly bent. Keeping your buttocks pressed against the wall, swing both legs up against the wall, settle your back on the floor, and rest your arms on the floor with your palms up. Align your body so your shoulders square up with your hips; your arms will angle out from your body alongside your hips. Hold for one to five minutes, as comfort allows. To come out of the pose, let your knees sink slowly toward your chest, and then roll to one side.

100 Stretch with a Bolster

Place a bolster, firm pillow, or rolled-up blanket on the floor and lie down on it so that it supports your upper back while the top of your head dangles back and touches the floor. (Make sure this angle is not too severe, especially if you have neck or back problems; you don't want to put any undue strain on your neck.) Keep your legs together, and gently drum your fingertips on your breastbone (the center of your chest) to stimulate your thymus gland, an important regulator in the body's immune system. Hold for about one minute, then use your arms to raise yourself into a sitting position.

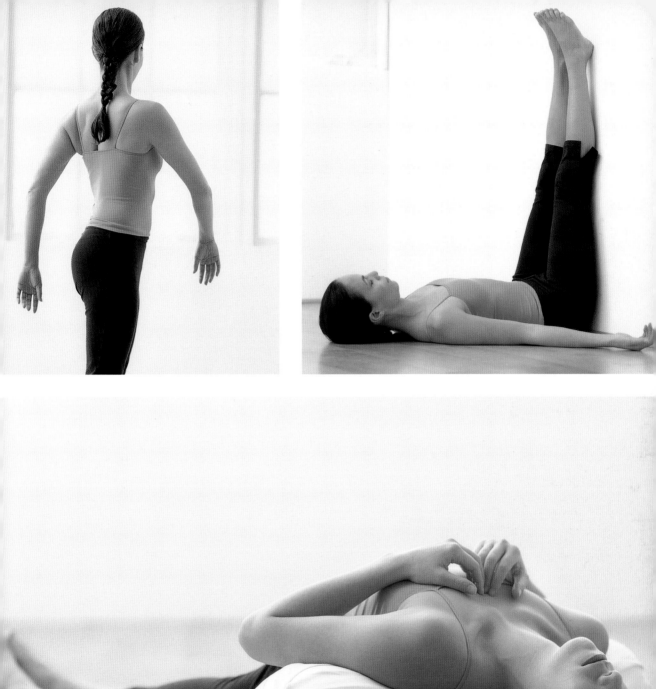
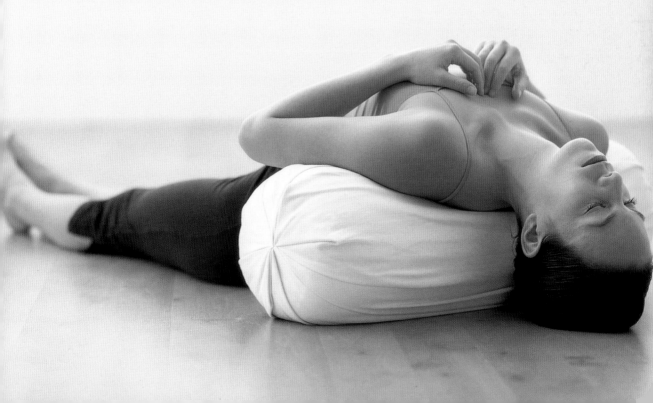

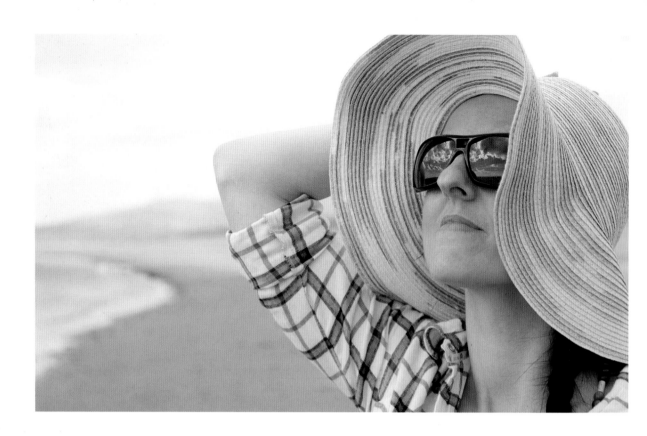

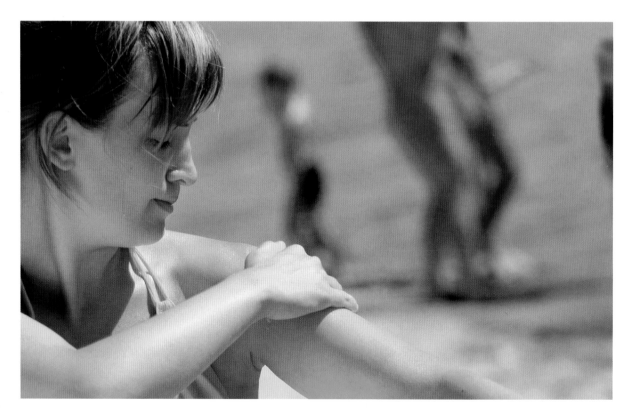

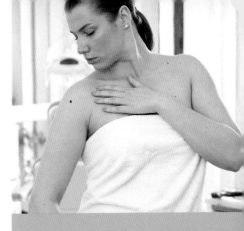

101 Stay Sun-Safe

We've all heard the message to wear sunblock every day, rain or shine, to prevent skin cancer and early wrinkles. However, if sunblock isn't yet part of your daily routine, you're far from alone, according to recent research. These tips on sun protection might help.

The best sunblock is the one that you will apply every day. It should offer UVA and UVB broad-spectrum protection, have an SPF of 30 or greater, and be water resistant, recommends the American Academy of Dermatology. Keep some in your purse, gym bag, car, office—anywhere and everywhere that's convenient. Consider multipurpose skin products, like a tinted moisturizer. Lotions and creams are easier to use on dry skin, gels on your scalp, and sticks around your eyes and on your lips.

Wear a wide-brimmed hat, wraparound sunglasses that block UVA and UVB, and clothing to protect exposed skin. Seek out shade when possible, and schedule outdoor activities before 10 AM or after 2 PM. If you want to look sun-kissed, use self-tanner. Do not use tanning beds! Indoor tanning before age 35 increases the risk of melanoma by a whopping 75 percent. Despite being a preventable risk factor for skin cancer, indoor tanning remains popular, especially with women 18 to 25, according to the Centers for Disease Control and Prevention.

102 Pour a Shot

A common pitfall when putting on sunblock is not using enough—most people apply only 25 to 50 percent of the recommended amount. You want to generously coat all of your exposed skin with a broad-spectrum, water-resistant sunblock that has an SPF of 30 or greater. That takes at least one ounce—enough to fill a shot glass.

103

Check Your Birthday Suit

Skin cancer is the most common form of cancer in the United States; melanoma is the most deadly type of skin cancer. However, skin cancer is very treatable when caught early. Get to know your own skin, so that you can recognize changes. Have your birthday serve as a reminder to give yourself a thorough annual self-exam. Make sure you have good light, and use a mirror to help you look everywhere, from behind your ears to between your toes. If you notice anything on your skin that is changing, growing, or bleeding, see a dermatologist.

104 Drink (Tea) to Your Health

Tea is the most popular beverage in the world after water. A simple cup of tea has long been used to warm the body and soothe the nerves, and many people instinctively reach for one when they're sick or feeling frazzled. Researchers now know that the brew also offers many health benefits, including preventing a variety of illnesses.

The leaves of black, green, white, and oolong teas (that is, any tea derived from the evergreen *Camellia sinensis*, which doesn't include herbal varieties) are rich in chemicals called polyphenols, which contain the antioxidants that may combat illnesses including heart disease and several types of cancer. The amino acid L-theanine, which is found in tea, boosts the body's defenses against bacterial, viral, fungal, and parasitic infections. Tea can protect against osteoporosis and some kinds of allergies. Iced and hot teas have equal amounts of antioxidants, but be aware that some ready-made, bottled teas can have low antioxidant levels and high sugar contents.

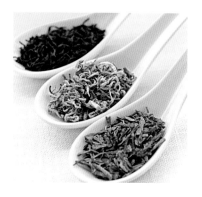

Choose Loose or Bagged

The health benefits are the same whether you use loose tea or tea bags. Steep your tea for at least three minutes to release antioxidants and other helpful substances.

Know Your Tea

The media's trumpeting of tea's many health benefits has resulted in an explosion of exotic varieties available in stores and online. But the differences among the main varieties can be confusing. Here's a quick guide to help you sort out your tea options.

TYPE	PROCESSING TECHNIQUE	CHARACTERISTICS
Black (also known as red tea)	Still-green leaves are withered, then rolled. Oxidation darkens leaves. Dried in ovens.	Flavors from nutty and spicy to flowery. Accounts for about 90 percent of tea consumption in the Western world.
Green	Leaves are allowed to wither, then are steamed or pan-fried, rolled, and dried. No oxidation.	Light, slightly bitter, grassy flavors. Most popular tea in Asia.
White	Leaves with white down are picked, steamed, and dried. No oxidation. Dried by pan-frying.	Delicate, complex, and sweet flavors. The rarest and most expensive tea.
Oolong	After withering, leaves are bruised and allowed to partially oxidize. Dried by pan-frying.	Fragrant and naturally sweet flavors. Properties are somewhere between the black and green teas.

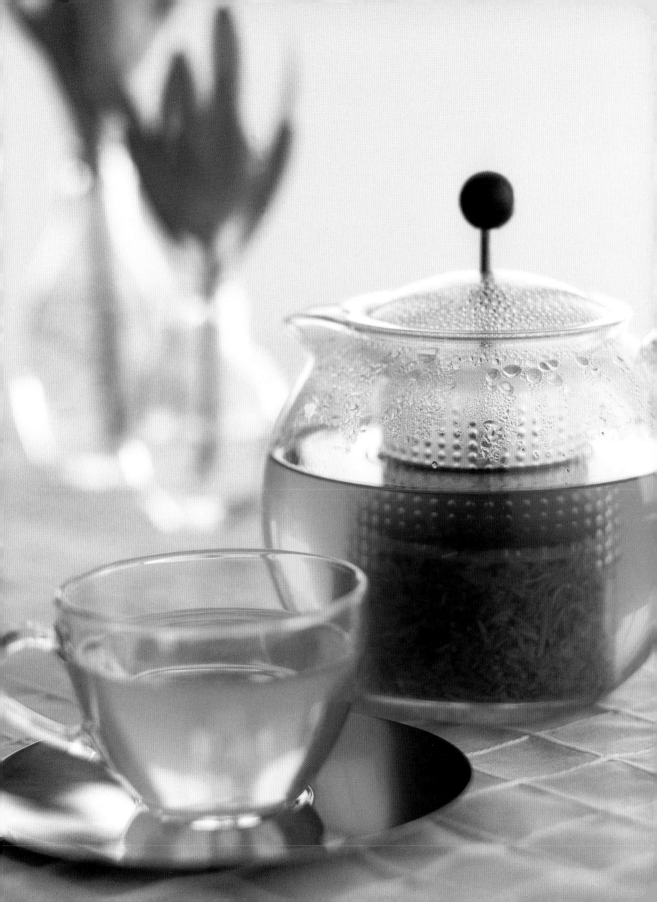

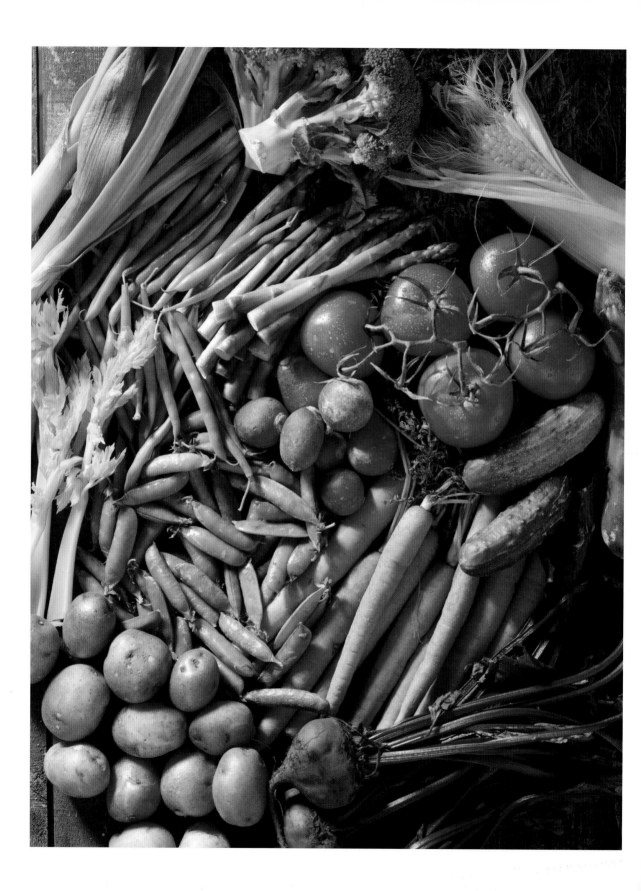

105 Clean (Up) Your Plate

While "clean-eating" is the current buzz, the reality is that it's pretty much the same rules we've been hearing for years: Avoid processed foods, stick to whole grains, limit "bad fats," eat as close to nature as possible, and have five or six small meals each day. As the noted author Michael Pollan distills it: "Eat food, not too much, mostly plants."

- Kick off your clean-eating plan at the grocery store. Stick to the perimeter of the store, where the fresh foods are sold. The goal is to buy organic foods in their natural state (whole fruits, vegetables, nuts, seeds) and avoid processed foods. Read labels! Clean eating involves fewer (and healthier) ingredients on the list. One rule of thumb is to never eat any packaged food that has more than five ingredients, or something that you can't identify.

- Eliminate refined sugar and products with added sugar. Use natural liquid sweetener, such as honey, agave, or maple syrup instead. Load up on "superfoods"—figs, avocados, local honey, blueberries, salmon, olive oil, brown rice, kale, sweet potatoes, Greek yogurt— the list goes on. Even if overhyped, each is packed with healthy nutrients.

- Keep the glycemic index (GI) of foods in mind. Foods with carbs that break down quickly and release glucose into the bloodstream right away, such as white flour, tend to have a high GI, while carbs that release glucose more gradually, such as whole grains, have a low GI. Generally speaking, lower-GI foods are the way to go: They're all-around healthier and make you feel full longer.

If you're coming from a processed-food diet and not loving the new flavors, keep in mind that your taste buds can adjust; give yourself time to acclimate. As you refine your approach to this new way of eating, you may encounter different philosophies—some allow low-fat dairy, for example, while others warn against it. Like any diet, figuring out what works for you is a process, so experiment with clean-eating principles and go with what makes you feel best.

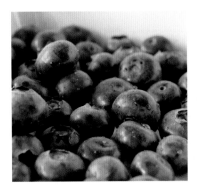

Pick Colorful Fruits

Most dietary guidelines recommend that plant-based foods—fresh fruits, vegetables, and whole grains—make up the bulk of what you eat. That's partly because they're high in fiber and nutrients, but it's also because they contain phytochemicals, naturally occurring substances that help boost the immune system and prevent or fight certain diseases. Dark red, blue, and purple vegetables and fruits— beets, blueberries, plums—are rich with phytochemicals. Just aim to eat a rainbow of foods; bright colors usually signal the presence of phytochemicals.

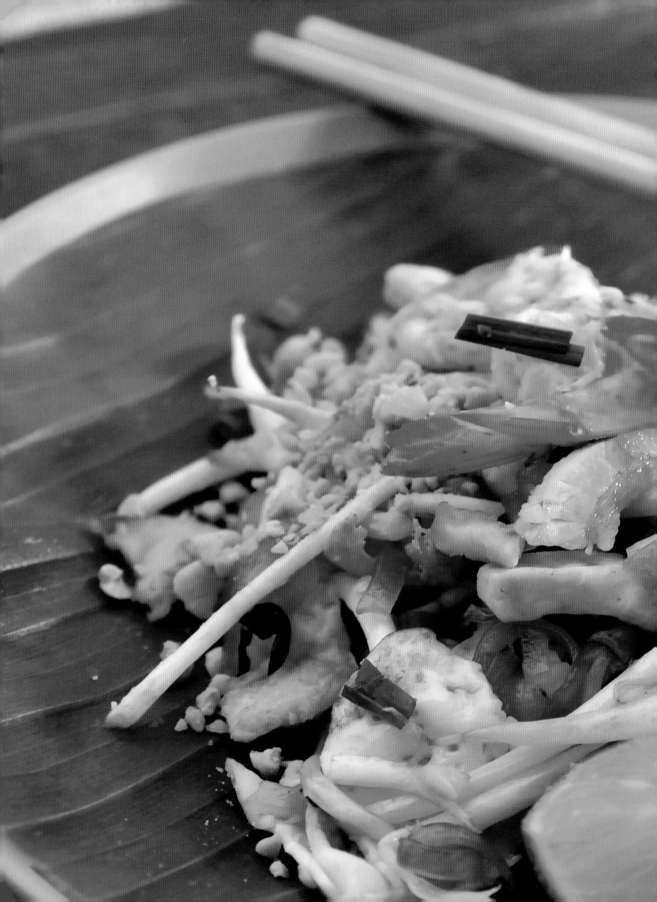

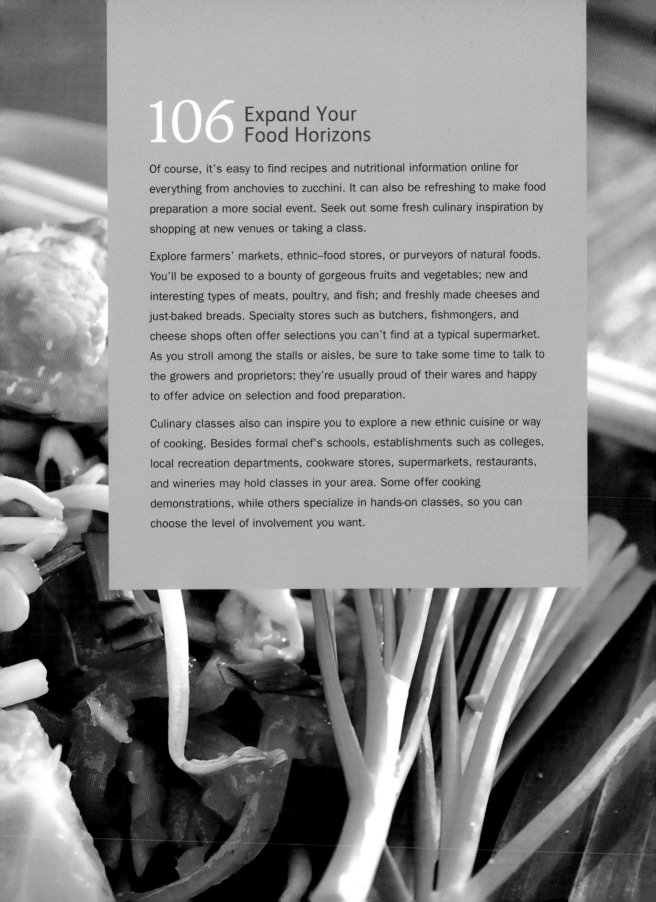

106 Expand Your Food Horizons

Of course, it's easy to find recipes and nutritional information online for everything from anchovies to zucchini. It can also be refreshing to make food preparation a more social event. Seek out some fresh culinary inspiration by shopping at new venues or taking a class.

Explore farmers' markets, ethnic–food stores, or purveyors of natural foods. You'll be exposed to a bounty of gorgeous fruits and vegetables; new and interesting types of meats, poultry, and fish; and freshly made cheeses and just-baked breads. Specialty stores such as butchers, fishmongers, and cheese shops often offer selections you can't find at a typical supermarket. As you stroll among the stalls or aisles, be sure to take some time to talk to the growers and proprietors; they're usually proud of their wares and happy to offer advice on selection and food preparation.

Culinary classes also can inspire you to explore a new ethnic cuisine or way of cooking. Besides formal chef's schools, establishments such as colleges, local recreation departments, cookware stores, supermarkets, restaurants, and wineries may hold classes in your area. Some offer cooking demonstrations, while others specialize in hands-on classes, so you can choose the level of involvement you want.

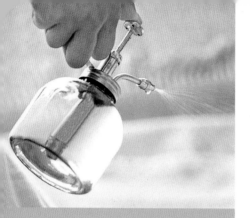

107
Soothe with Scent

For a little TLC during that time of the month, try aromatherapy. To help ease mood swings, scent your room using a spray-mister filled with ten drops of bergamot, lavender, or geranium essential oil and four ounces of water. To help relieve fluid retention, add five drops of patchouli or rosemary essential oil to two teaspoons of carrier oil, and massage yourself. To help quiet cramps, add two drops of clary sage or five drops of chamomile essential oil to a bowl of cool water, wet a towel, and put it on your abdomen.

108 Ease Period Pain with Yoga

Some women sail through their periods with nary a mood swing or cramp. Others aren't so lucky. To increase your comfort, find a place that's quiet and private, and try a simple and effective treatment aimed at lessening cyclical discomfort in your breasts, back, and belly.

1 If you're experiencing lower back pain, try doing a few knee circles. Lie on your back and bring your knees up toward your chest, keeping your back flat on the floor. Begin to make slow circles with your knees together, gently sweeping them across your abdomen from the right side to the left, continuing around for ten circles. Then repeat, circling ten times in the opposite direction.

2 Another good exercise for your back is to kowtow, sit back on your heels, and place your arms on the floor close to your body with the palms up. Rest your head on the floor and breathe slowly and deeply, trying to push your exhaled breath into your lower back. Repeat for five breaths, or until the pain subsides.

3 To help ease minor cramps, sit on the floor and bring the soles of your feet together. Grasp them with both hands; be careful not to pull up on your feet. Inhale fully and then lean forward slowly as you exhale, going only as far as feels comfortable while getting a good, gentle stretch in your back and waist. Hold for three to five breaths.

109 Ease Cramps with an Energy Hold

A simple exercise called an Energy Hold can help relieve menstrual cramps. To do this, lie on your back and rub your hands together vigorously until they feel warm. Now rest them on your abdomen, with your right hand below your navel and your left hand above it. Using your hands, gently rock your torso from side to side for about 20 seconds. Be still for 20 seconds, visualizing the warmth of your hands soothing any pain. Repeat, alternating rocking and stillness.

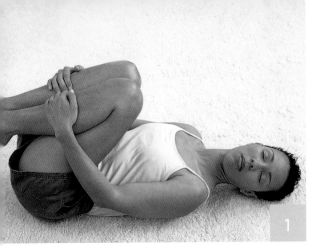

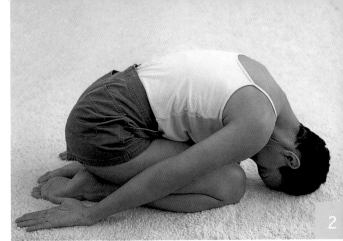

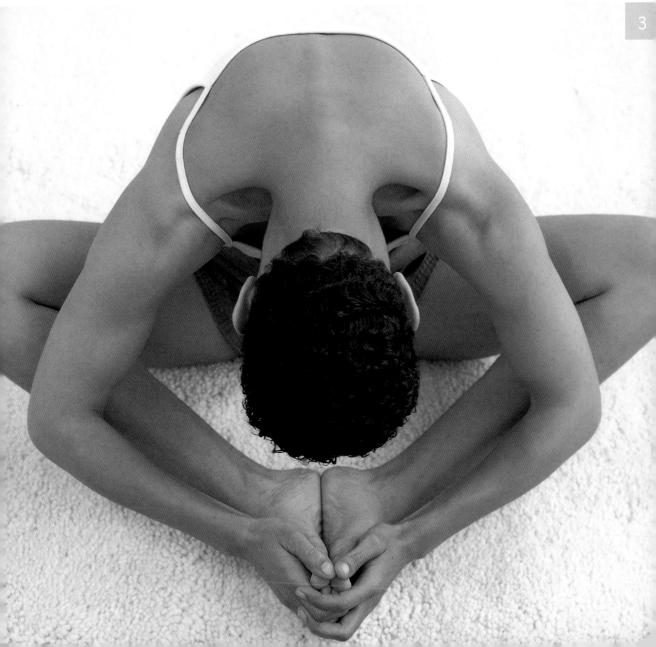

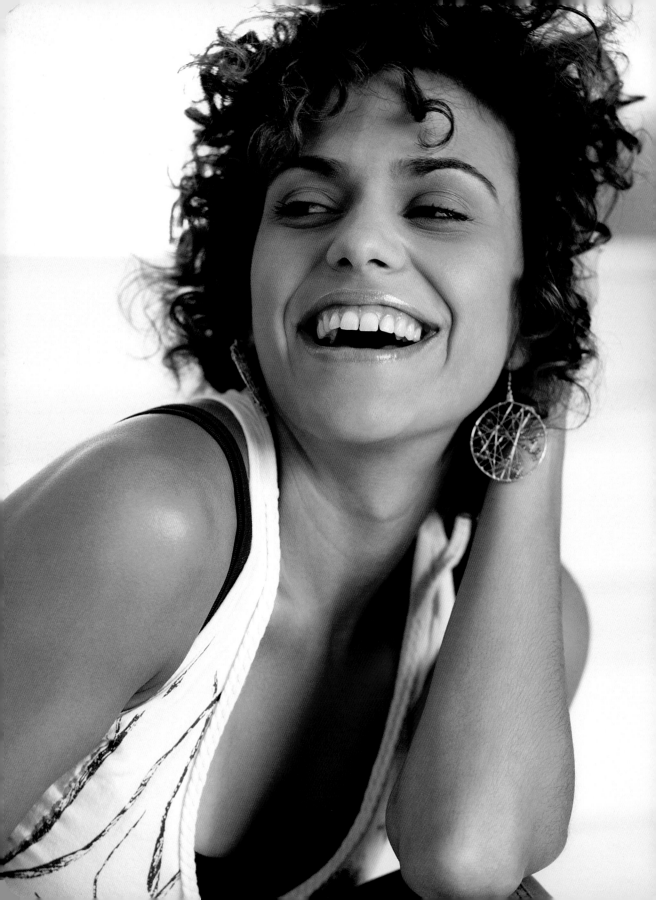

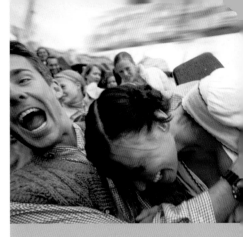

110 Come On, Get Happy

Happy people are healthier and live longer, according to research on the science of happiness. So what makes us happy? Family and relationships top the happiness-inducing list, which also includes positive thinking, meaningful work, gratitude, and the ability to forgive.

To raise your happiness quotient, make it a point to spend face-to-face time with friends and family by accepting social invitations and initiating easy-to-accomplish gatherings. Have neighbors over for ice cream, meet a friend for coffee, or take a lunchtime walk with a colleague. Yes, it's easier and faster to dash off an email or post a note online, but spending time with the people you love will make you happier. Physical contact, such as hugs, ups the ante by producing the bonding hormone oxytocin as well as feel-good endorphins.

Your attitude, which, unlike emotions, is something you can control, also has a profound effect on your happiness. Even if you're not feeling sunny, try to act as if you are, and the emotion will likely follow. When the going gets tough, positive thinking is especially important. In her groundbreaking research, psychologist Barbara Fredrickson has found that positive emotions are the most important element in determining a person's resilience in hard times. They help our bodies and our minds cope with stress, challenges, and negative feelings.

111 Love the Life You Have

People almost always overestimate the impact having more or less wealth will have on their happiness, according to researchers. In fact, the desire to have more money and material possessions often decreases happiness. The trick is to earn enough money to provide the essentials, be content with and grateful for what you have, and avoid comparing yourself to others. If you do compare, compare down. Olympic bronze medalists who consider themselves lucky to get a medal are happier than silver medalists who feel that they just missed the gold.

112 Have an Adventure

The same old dinner-and-a-movie routine can make a romantic relationship just as routine. To rev up romance, think novelty: Enjoying new and different activities together, especially ones that produce adrenaline (roller coaster, anyone?), will intensify your bond, according to researchers. Switching it up even a little (trying a new cuisine or film genre) will strengthen your connection.

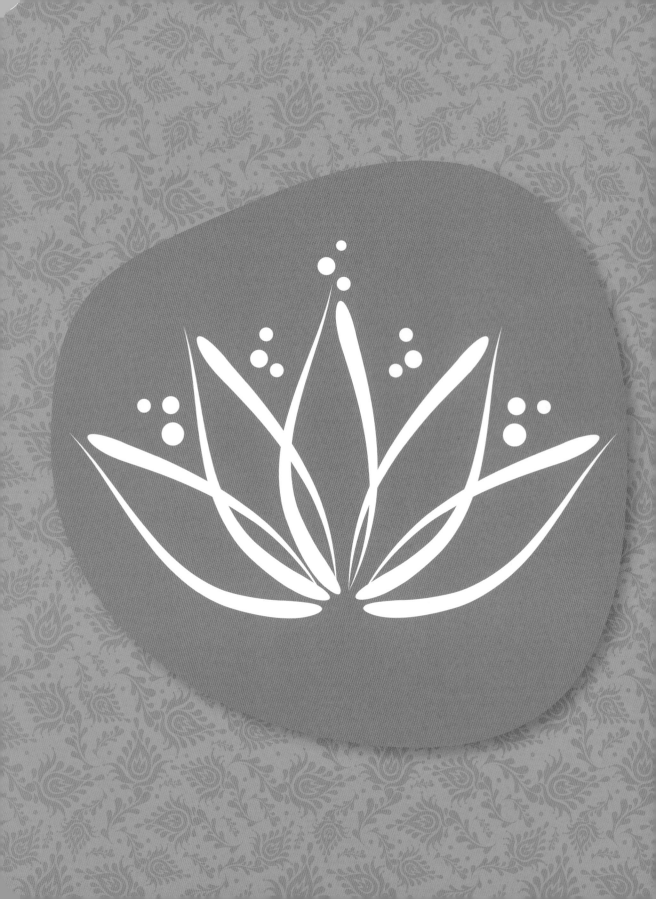

energize

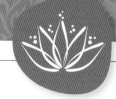

With all the things we'd like to do—let alone have to do—it's no wonder that few of us are able to breeze through the day with energy to spare. In fact, chronic fatigue is one of the most common complaints doctors hear. Often the energy-sapping culprits are lifestyle factors such as too little sleep, overscheduling, and, above all, stress.

While you can't add more hours to the day, you can rethink your work, family, and social commitments, and learn to say no to the ones that are less pleasurable or pressing. If a lack of sleep is your downfall, the solution is obvious—get more of it—but, in the real world, that can be hard to do. If you're feeling stressed—the number one cause of chronic fatigue—the exercises, treatments, and activities in this chapter are guaranteed to help you handle everyday stress better and put a little more zip in your step. ✎

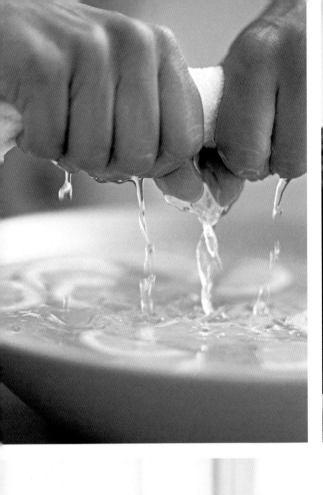
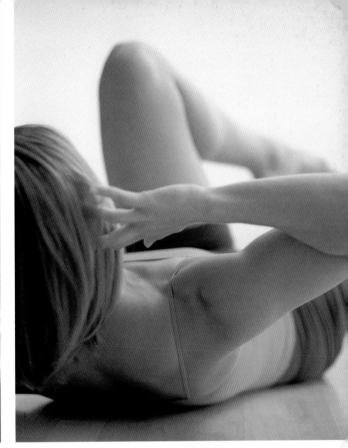
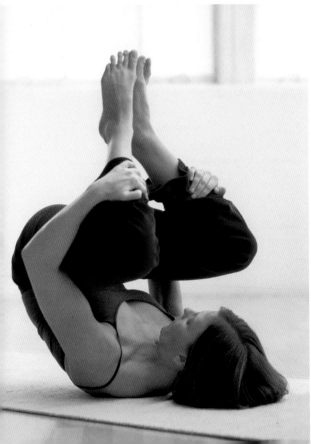
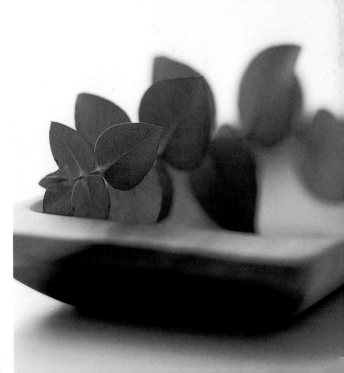

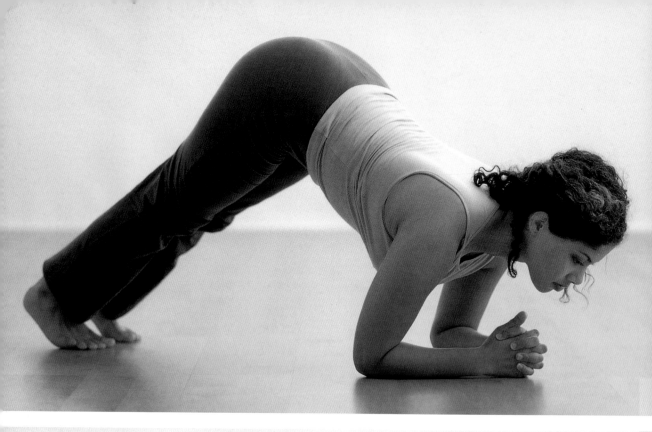

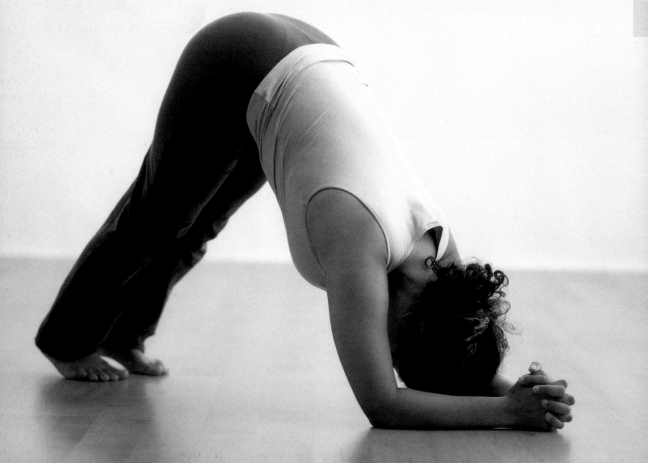

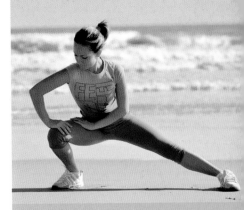

113 Get Strong Shoulders with Dolphin Pose

The challenging Dolphin pose, reminiscent of the graceful arc of a dolphin's body, builds upper-body strength and provides a pleasant stretch for the back muscles that run along your spine. It also promotes neck strength, which is vital for preparing for headstands and other demanding poses.

1 To get into position, kneel down and grasp each of your upper arms with the opposite hand. Then, still grasping your upper arms, place your elbows on the floor. Keeping your elbows where they are, release your hands and interlace your fingers; lower your forearms to the floor. Make sure that your elbows are slightly closer together than your shoulders are. Next, simultaneously press down with your arms, as if you're trying to push the floor away from your chest, and lift your hips as pictured. Lengthen your spine and allow your head to hang down. Keeping your back straight, inhale and extend your head past your hands, reaching forward with your chin.

2 Exhale and press your chest toward your feet so that your head comes inside your arms. Let your neck relax. Move back and forth between the positions as many times as your comfort level allows.

114 Find Your Inner Flexibility

It's tempting to think that you're fit if you're strong and in good aerobic shape. But be sure to also work on flexibility, the third leg of any fitness program. Muscles that are short or stiff are more prone to injury, as are the joints near those muscles. On the other hand, lengthened muscles and joints with a good range of motion (both of which come from stretching) withstand trauma more easily and perform better in both competitive sports and daily activities.

115 Time Your Stretches

To get the most out of static stretching, give your muscles the time they need to let go:

- Warm up with at least five to ten minutes of aerobic activity, which can be as simple as brisk walking.

- Gently stretch to the point of tension, never pain, and then hold for 30 seconds to two minutes. Look at your watch—this often will feel like a long time!

- Breathe deeply and try to focus on releasing muscle tension during exhales. Make your exhales longer than your inhales.

- Do not bounce. Strive for a gentle, sustained stretch, breathing through areas of resistence until they naturally release. Never force a stretch.

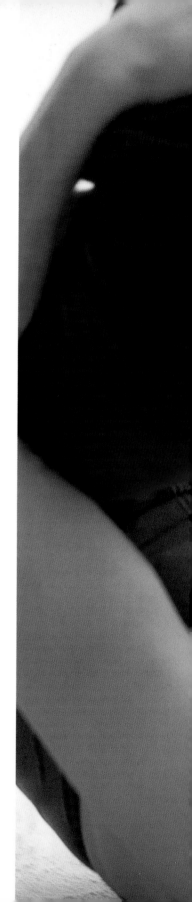

116 Feel the Power of Pilates

Sure, you can turn to lattes and chocolate croissants for a rush of morning energy. But the highs you get from caffeine and sugar can first make you jittery and then leave you tired. Instead, jump-start your day with a healthy breakfast and some exercise. Exercising can fend off fatigue and brighten your morning outlook. Beginning your day with a short Pilates workout (see following pages) will clarify your mind and loosen your body.

Pilates exercises are based on the original work of Joseph Pilates, a German who deeply believed in the importance of mental and physical conditioning. The system of slow, focused exercises he developed is designed to elongate the body, increase flexibility, strengthen muscles, and focus the mind.

Over time, practicing Pilates can help you develop more sustained energy. Strong muscles moving freely (that is, not bound by pain or stiffness) naturally impart more energy. And a calm mind (one not jangled by stress) naturally feels much clearer.

117 Balance Back and Ab Muscles

Your back muscles stabilize your spinal column, allowing you to stand upright and bend and straighten your body. They provide support for your chest and extra power for your arms. These muscles also work in concert with your abdominal muscles to assist in breathing and protect your internal organs. To maintain a balance between the two muscle groups, pair back-strengthening poses with ab exercises.

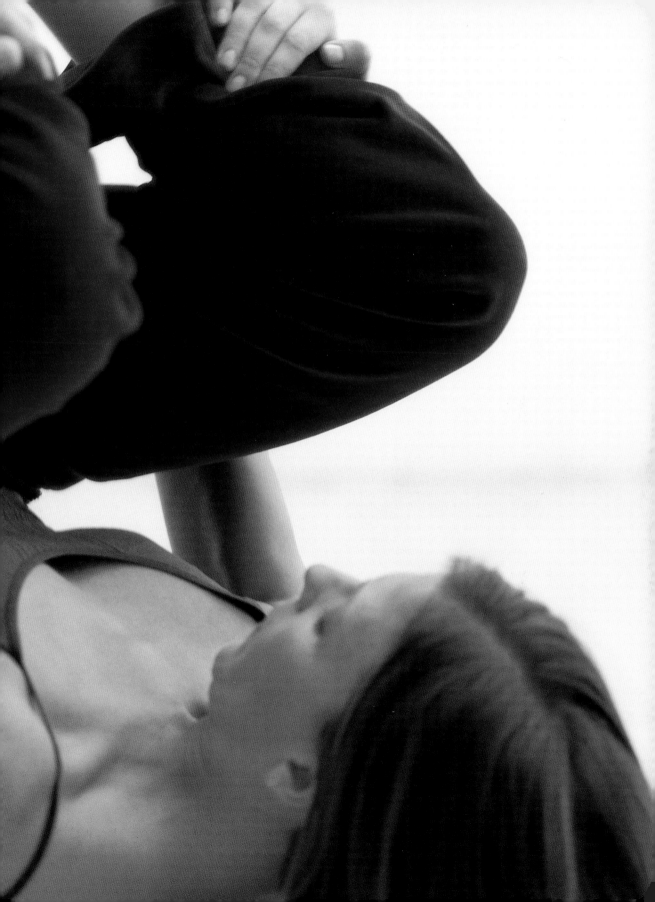

118 Try Basic Pilates Moves

Strengthen and loosen your body with this Pilates workout. Doing it in the morning will help you feel focused, flexible, and ready to start the day with some pep.

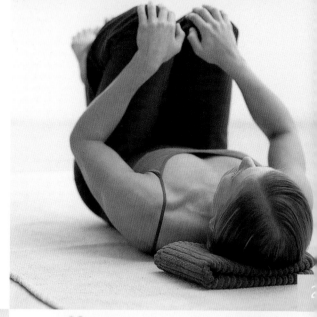

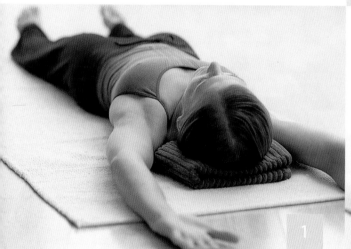

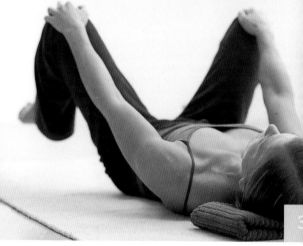

1 To begin, lie on your back on a mat or other comfortably padded surface; if you like, you can use a folded towel as a pillow to cushion your head. Keep your legs hip-width apart, your arms stretched out way overhead, and your fingers spread wide. Push through the balls of your feet so that you lengthen your spine, but don't arch your back.

2 Bend your knees, positioning your thighs perpendicular to the floor while your lower legs dangle. Place your hands on top of your knees. Maintain a little space between the floor and the small of your back.

3 Lightly pressing your palms down on your knees, circle your legs away from each other, down away from the torso, and around back together. While your legs are moving, try to keep your pelvis steady. Circle eight times, then eight times in the other direction.

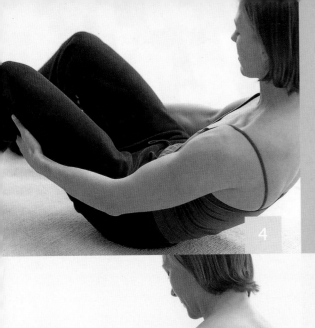

Kick off your day with this short Pilates workout designed to help you feel focused, flexible, and ready to go. Follow with a healthy breakfast with whole grains, low-fat protein, low-fat dairy, and fruits and vegetables—a combo that combines complex carbohydrates, fiber, and protein—and will keep you fueled for hours.

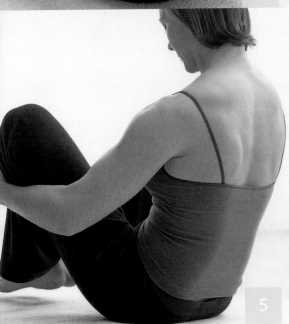

4 With your legs bent and your hands on the backs of your thighs, slowly roll up using your abdominal muscles. Slowly roll back down to the ground, rounding your back and pressing the back of your rib cage to the floor. Roll back up. Repeat eight times.

5 Roll up and sit with your feet on or off the floor (use whichever position is easier for you). If they're off the floor, balance on your buttocks.

6 Tighten your abdominals, round your lower back, open your knees, and hold on to the front of your shins with your hands. Keep your elbows wide and your chin slightly tucked in. Staying rounded in a little ball, rock back and forth on your back. Avoid rocking onto your neck. Focus on inhaling as you rock backward and exhaling as you rock forward. Repeat eight times.

119 Rev Up with an Invigorating Massage

Not all massages are meant to soothe. The brisk motions used in this massage are perfect for revving up before a workout or a demanding day at work. Recruit a friend to give you this invigorating massage treatment, which is particularly ideal when you're under a lot of stress. Begin the massage lying facedown on a firm, comfortable surface, and ask your friend to follow these four steps:

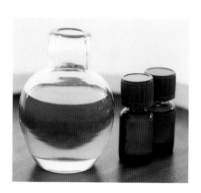

Energizing Massage Blend

2 ounces carrier oil
16 drops geranium essential oil
7 drops rosemary essential oil
2 drops peppermint essential oil

1 Warm some massage oil (see the recipe at left) between your palms and spread a light, even layer across your friend's back and sides. Starting at the waist, press your hands up along each side of her spine, gliding to the top. Fan your hands out across her shoulders, draw your fingers down along her ribs and sides, and pull your hands back to her waist. Keep your hands and fingers relaxed and molded to the contours of her body. Apply more pressure as you stroke up, less as you stroke down. Continue for several minutes.

2 With your friend faceup or facedown, spread massage oil evenly onto one leg. Using gliding motions, encircle as much of her leg as possible. Lead the stroke with the web of your hand (the skin between the thumb and index finger). Start at the ankle and move over the calf and thigh using firm pressure (use light pressure on the knee); glide back toward her ankle with lighter pressure. Stroke slowly, then speed up for two minutes. Repeat on the other leg.

3 Lift one of her hands, and firmly glide your other hand from her wrist to elbow to arm socket; glide lightly back to the wrist. Lead the stroke with the web of your cupped hand. Establish a brisk pattern for about one minute. Repeat on the other arm.

4 Knead her back. Work smaller muscles with your thumb and fingertips in a gentle motion like a cat's paw opening and closing in contentment. Push and pull larger muscles with wider, deeper movements, as if kneading dough. Continue for a few minutes.

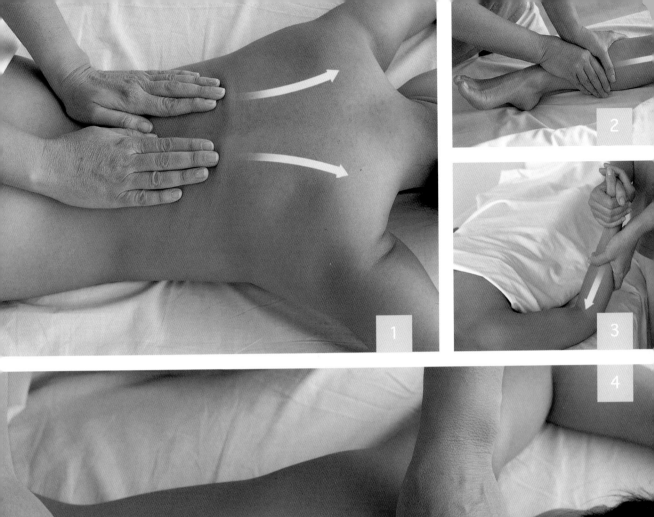

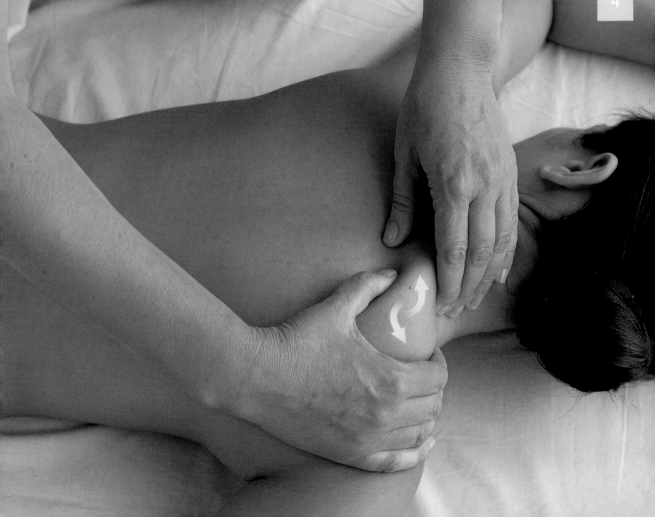

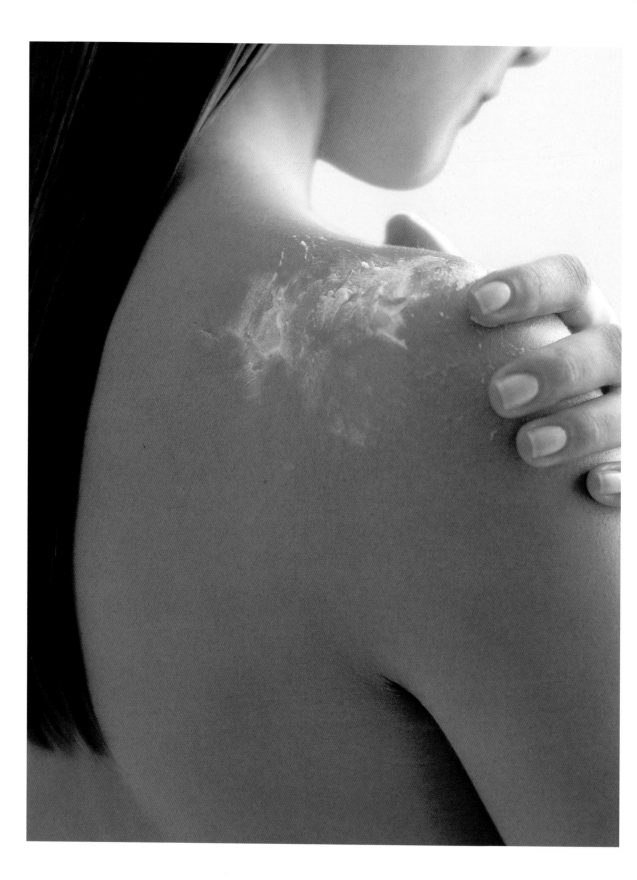

120 Moisturize with Stimulating Eucalyptus Lotion

After your shower, take time for a step that can make a big difference to the rest of your day: Moisturize, from top to toes, using a product with a refreshing scent, such as eucalyptus.

Take a warm, brief shower and dry off lightly, leaving your skin slightly damp. This traps some of the moisture in your skin when you apply the body lotion. Starting with your shoulders and working downward, apply a liberal amount of moisturizer, rubbing it in well and putting a little extra on dry patches of skin.

The scent you choose can have a big effect on your mood, and if it's energy you're craving, eucalyptus (pictured at right) simply can't be beat. Its bracing aroma is a wake-up call for the mind; its chemical components act as both a deodorant and stimulant for the body. If the scent doesn't appeal to you, explore other energizing essential oils such as rosemary, cypress, bay laurel, basil, lemon, or orange.

You can use a preformulated product or just add a few drops of eucalyptus essential oil—or a blend of oils (see recipe at right)—to an unscented moisturizer. You're not limited to lotion here; there are many different types of moisturizers. If your skin is very dry, a scented oil, a body butter, or a cream moisturizer will leave it feeling soft and well hydrated. If your skin is normal, either a cream or an emollient-rich body lotion probably will do the trick. If your skin is oily or prone to pimples, stick to a lighter body lotion, making sure that it's noncomedogenic (which means that it won't clog pores).

You'll find hundreds of choices, so you may need to experiment to find the one that has just the right scent and feel for you. Take advantage of testers in stores, keeping in mind that products that seem overly greasy, sticky, or thick in the jar or tube might melt wonderfully into your skin once applied. Also notice which ones have staying power; some will keep your thirsty skin feeling hydrated much longer than others.

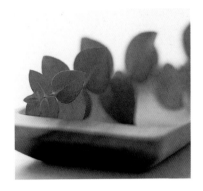

Bracing Body Lotion

2 ounces unscented lotion
10 drops eucalyptus essential oil
7 drops rosemary essential oil
5 drops pine essential oil
3 drops lemongrass essential oil

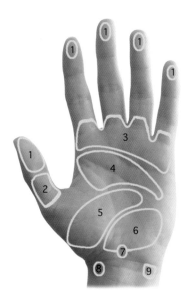

Left-Hand Reflexology Points

Here are some of the key reflexology points on the palm side of your left hand:

1 Sinus, head, and brain
2 Neck and throat
3 Eye and ear
4 Lung, breast, back, and heart
5 Stomach and pancreas
6 Intestines
7 Bladder
8 Uterus
9 Ovary

121 Zone In on Hand Reflexology

Human bodies have zones of energy, according to reflexologists, who recommend activating these zones to improve health and enhance feelings of well-being. Reflexology involves applying firm pressure to specific points on the hands and feet to exert influence on other body parts, organs, glands, and systems. The theory is that these reflexology points are linked by neurological and energy pathways to specific and often far-removed parts of the body. Pressure on a given point is thought to clear any energy blockages and to have either a stimulating or relaxing effect. All you need is a reflexology map (see the illustration at left) to guide you to the pertinent points on your hands.

1 To awaken your internal organs in the morning, stimulate their reflexology points by pressing the thumb of one of your hands deeply into the palm of your other hand. Move your thumb in little circles from the bottom of the palm to the base of each finger. (Another method is to position your thumb in the center of the palm and rock the palm onto the tip of your thumb. Then rock the palm off the thumb, move your thumb to a new position, and repeat the sequence.) Make sure that you cover the palm's entire surface. Steady, direct pressure is used to help reduce pain, while pressing and releasing (often called alternating pressure) helps stimulate the point. When you identify a body part that seems to warrant particular attention, try working its corresponding reflexology point for at least 30 seconds.

2 To stimulate energy in the reflexology zones in your sinuses, head, brain, neck, and throat, firmly press and circle the tip of each finger and the length of the thumb. Work both hands.

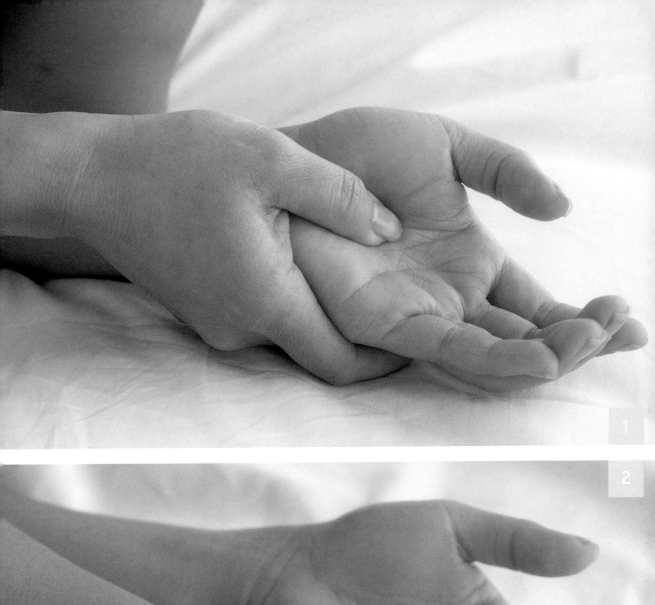

1

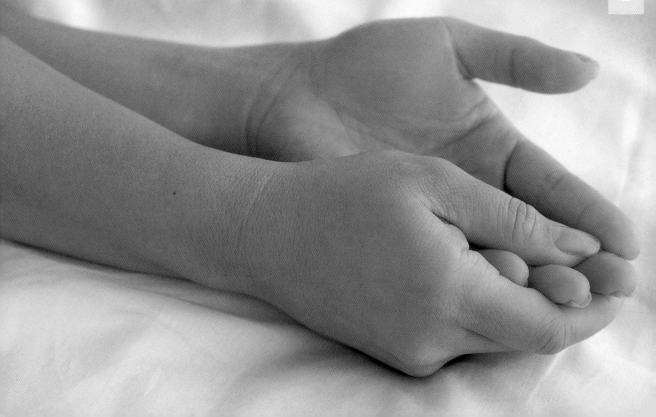

2

122 Bend Your Back into Cobra Pose

Backward-bending yoga poses, like Cobra, build strength, exert gentle pressure on the adrenal glands, and allow you to breathe more deeply, bestowing a sense of vigor. Lie facedown. Set your feet hip-width apart and point your toes. Resting your forehead on the floor, place your palms flat on the floor directly beneath your shoulders, bringing your elbows in toward your ribs. Inhale and gently extend your chin forward as you lift your head, neck, and chest as high as you can comfortably without putting pressure on your palms. Keep your shoulder blades low. Hold the pose for four to ten breaths, then release.

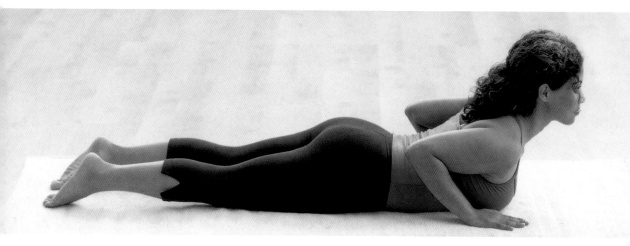

123 Get A.M. Energy with Ayurveda

To feel more energized in the morning, Ayurvedic yogis recommend a variety of practices that go far beyond starting the day with a yoga routine. They involve everything from the hour you rise to what you eat for breakfast. Ayurveda, the traditional medicine of India, is a centuries-old holistic health-care system. In Sanskrit, *ayur* means "life" and *veda* means "knowledge." The system teaches how to balance our life energies and achieve harmony with the environment, returning us to a natural state of health and happiness.

Ayurvedic eye-openers:

- Rise at least 20 minutes before the sun does.

- Splash cool water on your face seven times.

- Drink a glass of lukewarm water garnished with a lemon or lime slice.

- Use a tongue scraper, gently moving it from the back of the tongue to the front.

- Tap your teeth together to stimulate the *nadis*, channels through which energy flows.

124 Challenge Your Body with Bow Pose

Bow pose is a more challenging backward-bending yoga pose. Lie facedown on the floor, bend your knees, and bring your heels toward your hips; reach back to grasp your feet or ankles, whichever position is more comfortable. Allow your legs to separate, but keep your heels over your buttocks. Inhale, and raise your head, neck, chest, and thighs, pressing your feet into your hands and lifting your heels away from your back. Dont't strain—the quality of your effort is more important than how far your legs or chest lift up. Hold for four to six breaths. While exhaling, slowly lower yourself back down to the floor.

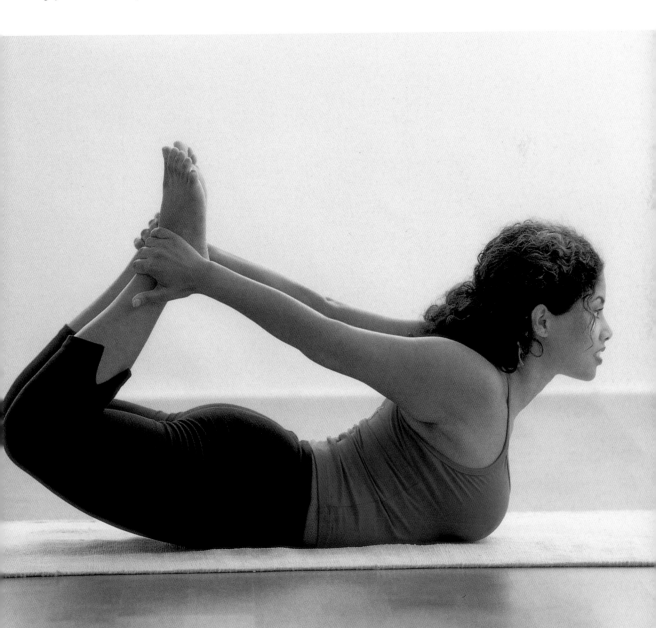

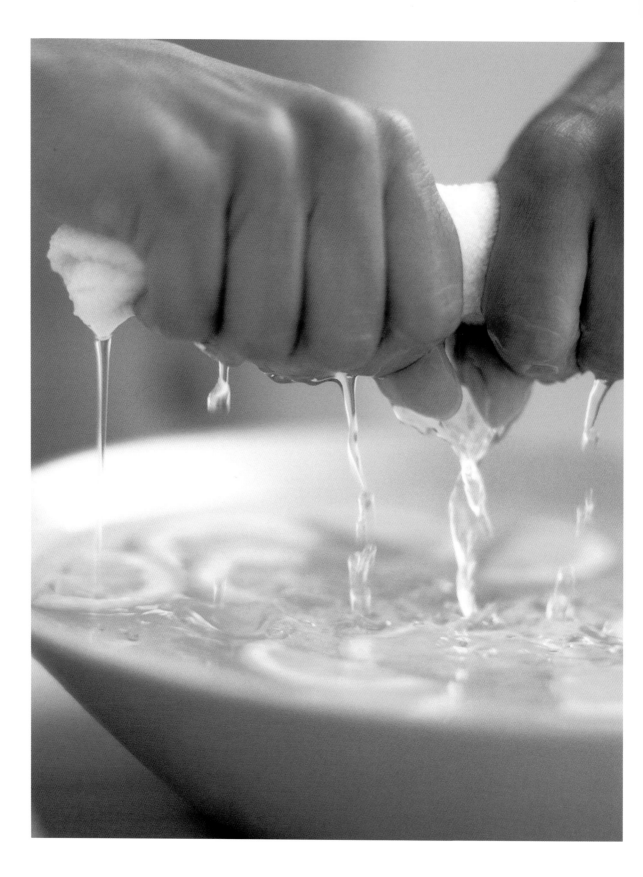

125 Increase Alertness with a Fresh Lemon Scrub

Aromatherapists say that lemon, with its fresh and bracing scent, is one of the most beneficial essential oils for stimulating the mind and increasing alertness. Start off your day with this refreshing treatment or simply try it as a pick-me-up before going out on the town.

Add lemon essential oil and fresh lemon slices to a small bowl of warm water (see recipe at right). Place a clean washcloth in the bowl to soak, allowing it to become infused with lemon oil. After a couple of minutes, swipe the cloth over any remaining oil droplets floating on top of the water, then wring it out.

Place the cloth within easy reach and run a warm shower (if you make it too hot, it will make you feel listless, not invigorated). Briefly cleanse your body, using a citrus-scented soap if possible, and rinse off thoroughly. After turning off the shower, fold the washcloth into a compact square and begin scrubbing your body with it. Start at your feet and move upward, always scrubbing toward your heart, which helps stimulate your circulatory system. Towel off, and keep that fresh feeling going by applying a citrus-scented body moisturizer.

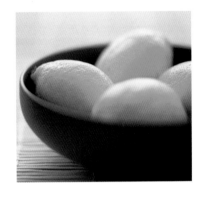

Fresh Lemon Scrub

5 drops lemon essential oil
6 or more fresh lemon slices
Small bowl of warm water
Washcloth
Citrus-scented soap (optional)
Citrus-scented body moisturizer

126 Wake Up to Lemon's Skin-Care Benefits

Lemons contain generous amounts of vitamin C, which is a powerful antioxidant, as well as healthy helpings of citric acid and vitamins A and B1. These helpful components encourage the exfoliation of dead skin, stimulate circulation, balance overactive oil glands, and help brighten the complexion. In a pinch, dilute lemon juice with water to make an effective toner.

127 Gather Energy with Tai Chi

Tai chi practitioners believe that you can increase the amount of chi, life's vital energy, in your body by gathering it from the air and the universe.

Chi is believed to come from a variety of sources. We inherit a kind of chi called *jing* from our parents. Other chi comes from the food we eat: Wholesome food possesses more chi than unhealthy food. Chi also comes from the air we breathe (the less polluted the better). Finally, some of our chi is derived from the universe itself. To gather chi:

1 Stand tall, with tailbone tucked in, knees gently bent, chin slightly down, feet shoulder-width apart, and arms hanging down, relaxed.

2 As you slowly squat, bring your arms out to create a large circle, as if you're about to pick up a beach ball. Make sure your elbows, wrists, and knees stay relaxed, your arms are rounded and wide, and your hands never quite touch each other as you gather up the ball.

3 Stand up again and, as you rise, bring your arms in toward your abdomen, as if you're trying to push the air out of the ball.

4 Now look up and raise your arms, keeping them rounded, as if reaching for another ball. Then bring your arms in toward your waist again, as if trying to deflate the ball. Drop your hands to your sides, and repeat the steps for three to five minutes.

128 Discover the Seven Chakras

In tai chi, yoga, and Eastern medicine, the body's *prana* (life force) is believed to flow along energy channels that intersect at chakras (or wheels), which are associated with distinct states of mind. The objective is to keep the chakras open, promoting physical, emotional, mental, and spiritual balance.

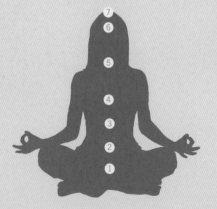

CHAKRA	LOCATION	ASSOCIATED WITH
First	Base of spine	Security, well-being
Second	Just beneath navel	Sensuality, fertility
Third	Solar plexus	Personal power, belonging
Fourth	Heart	Love, generosity
Fifth	Throat	Creativity, communication
Sixth	Between eyebrows	Intuition, awareness
Seventh	Top of head	Spirituality

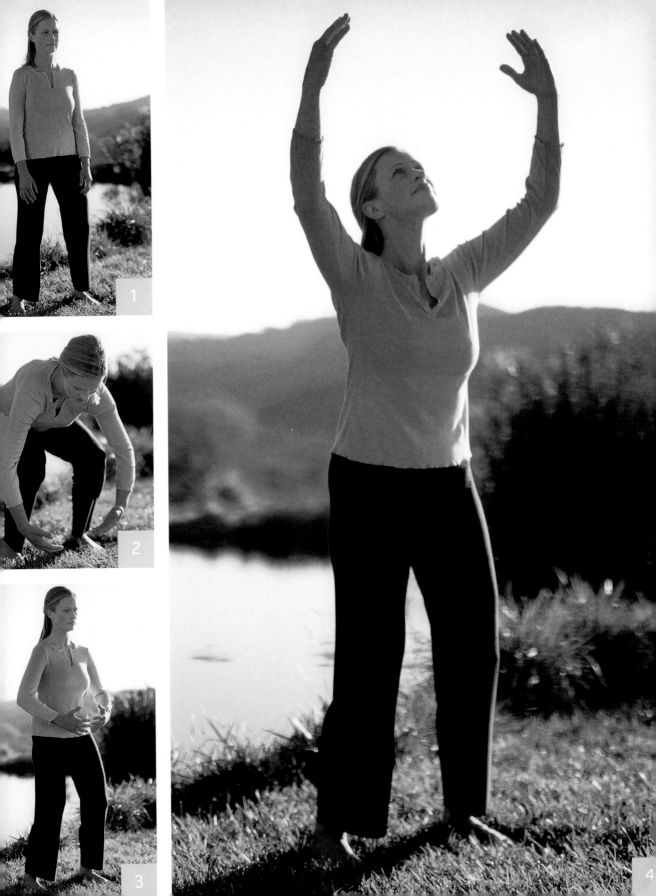

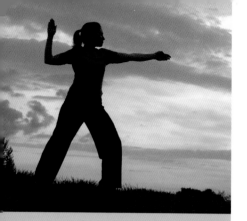

129

Move with Energy

Perform tai chi at a leisurely pace. Doing the gentle, flowing motions oh-so-slowly still gets your heart pumping, your limbs loosened, your mind engaged, and your whole body working. Also, as a form of moving meditation, tai chi is extremely helpful in relieving stress, the most potent energy zapper out there.

130 Encourage Energy Flow with the Opening Tai Chi Sequence

The Opening tai chi sequence encourages the flow of chi (life energy) throughout the body. Focus on keeping your body relaxed, joint angles soft, and mind focused. Usually done at the start of a tai chi session, it can also be practiced on its own for a stimulating effect.

1 With your eyes closed, spine straight, and feet close together, begin to clear your mind of thoughts and worries. Concentrate on the idea of gathering energy in your body. Breathe deeply and naturally. Spend a minute or two just quieting your mind and concentrating on awakening your dormant energy.

2 Open your eyes and step out to the side with one foot so your feet are shoulder-width apart; let your arms simply hang loosely at your sides. Imagine your weight settling down toward the earth.

3 Leading with your wrists, float your arms up to shoulder height, with the elbows and wrists slightly bent, palms facing in and fingers pointing down. Throughout the sequence, keep your shoulders dropped and relaxed and your legs relaxed and still. Tuck in your tailbone (you don't want your butt to stick out) and keep your chin slightly down.

4 Move down into a shallow squat—keep your knees softly bent, with your toes pointed forward and the knees positioned directly above your toes. As you begin to squat, lead with your wrists and allow your elbows to sink and your forearms to float up, with your fingers pointing up and your palms facing out.

5 As you rise, let your elbows flow up again and let your hands drop back down. Repeat the up-and-down motions eight times. Think about maintaining good mental and physical form as you flow up and down.

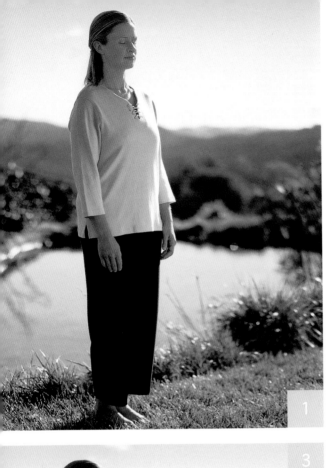

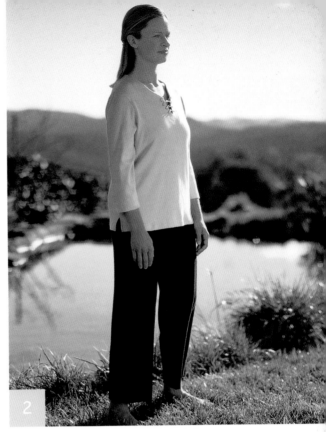

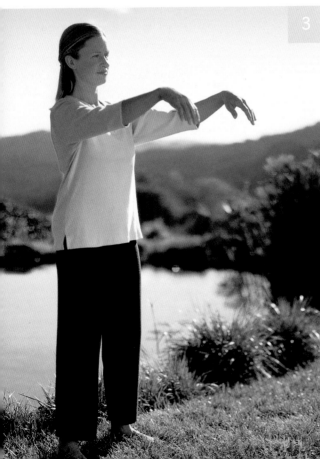

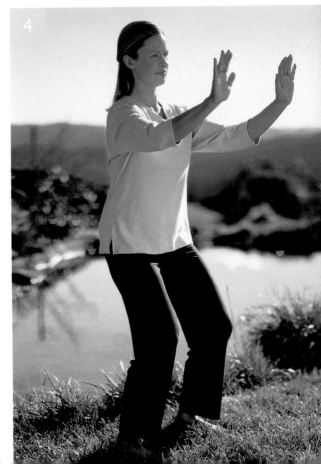

1

2

3

4

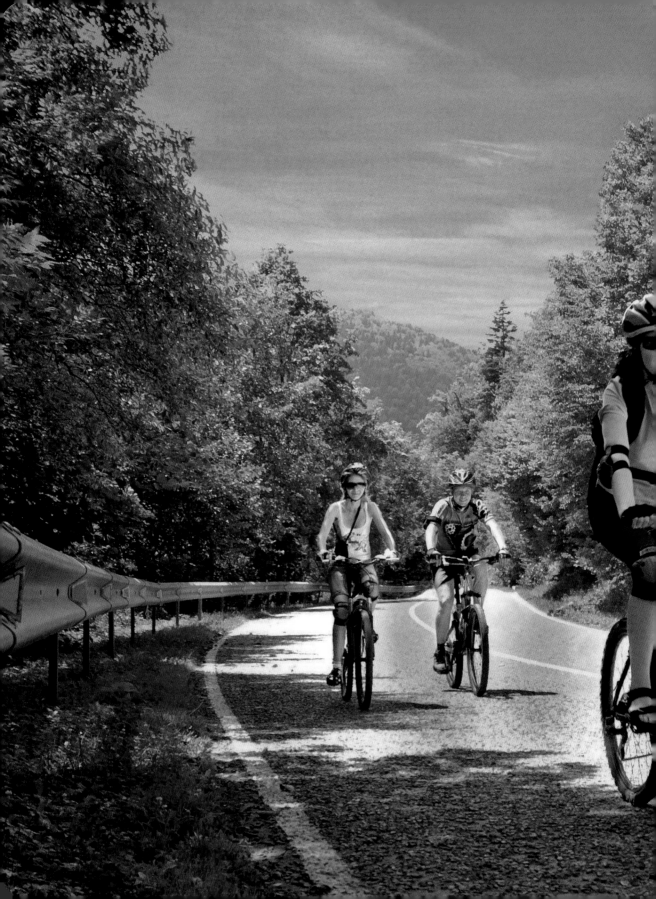

131 Go Outside and Play

Maybe the elliptical machine has become your cardio default, you've mastered the barre routine, or you feel the burn from a buff-your-bum podcast. But nothing revitalizes an exercise routine or provides a treat for mind and body like getting into the great outdoors for a vigorous workout.

The options are numerous, and, with a little experimentation, you're sure to find the right one for you. Maybe it's hiking nearby trails, swimming laps in a local pool, or joining a running group. Maybe it's time to dust off your bike, in-line skates, or skateboard (remember to always wear a helmet). Take your tai chi routine to a park, sign up for those sailing lessons you've always talked about, or go for walks around the neighborhood.

Make the most of the season. Play beach volleyball, or go snowboarding. Don't let chilly weather serve as an excuse to keep you inside; you actually burn around 5 percent more calories when you exercise in the cold, because your body has to work harder to maintain its core temperature—more bang for your exercise buck. (Whatever the temperature, be sure to stay hydrated.) No matter what form of outdoor activity you choose, you're sure to find that fresh air and fresh scenery result in a fresh attitude.

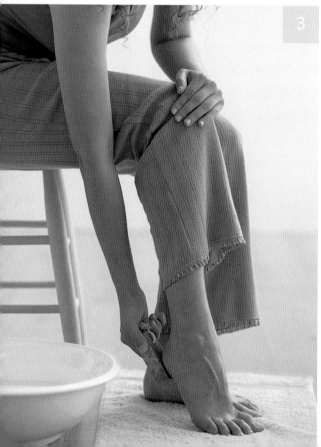
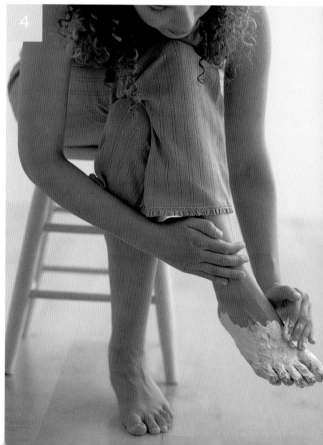
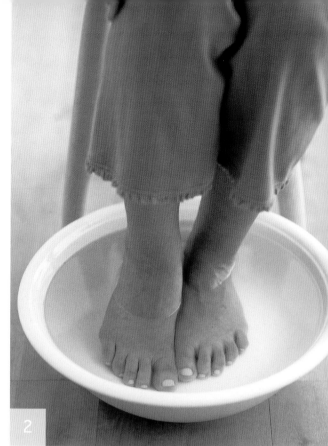
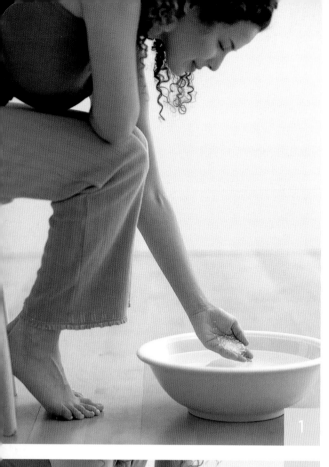

1 2 3 4

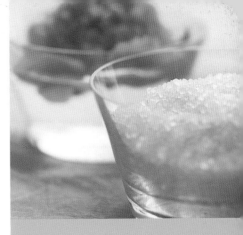

132 Dip into a Minty-Fresh Foot Bath

Powered by one of the most versatile and refreshing aromatic oils, this invigorating peppermint-oil foot treatment is a sure bet for putting a new bounce in your step.

1 Fill a large bowl with warm water, making sure that the water level will fall just below your ankles. Add one heaping tablespoon of peppermint oil mineral crystals to the water.

2 Soak your feet for at least ten minutes to soften and refresh your skin. Aside from being immensely soothing, the foot bath will make the next step—exfoliation—easier and more effective.

3 After thoroughly drying your feet, use a pumice stone to smooth out any rough patches on your heels. Firmly rub the stone up and down from the back of your heel to the bottom of your foot. Continue until the skin feels smoother. Repeat on the other foot.

4 If you have a little more time, follow up with a hydrating and energizing foot mask. Spread a thick layer of the mask over the tops and soles of your feet and in between your toes. Apply gently, and don't rub in. Leave on for 15 minutes, then thoroughly remove the mask by wiping with a wet washcloth or rinsing in the bathtub.

133 Know Your Bath Products

Confused by all the different formulations of bath products? Here's a cheat sheet. *Bath salts* typically are made from sea salt and essential oils or other fragrances; they help soften the skin and reputedly draw toxins from the body. *Bath foams* create bubbles, release pleasant scents, and can serve as a substitute for soap. *Bath oils,* which generally contain essential oils or other fragrances suspended in a light carrier oil, moisturize your skin. *Bath* (or *shower*) *gels* are a kind of liquid soap. *Bath teas* are tea bags filled with dried herbs purported to have a variety of therapeutic effects when left to steep in bathwater. Experiment and pick whichever ones feel and smell good to you.

134

Feel the Power of Peppermint

Drink peppermint tea to soothe an upset stomach, or smell its aroma to wake up. This popular medicinal plant is also credited with relieving headaches, acting as a nasal decongestant, and being a mental stimulant. Peppermint's prime active component is menthol. When applied to the skin, menthol quickly produces a cooling sensation, which the body reacts to by increasing blood flow to the area, creating a comforting sense of warmth.

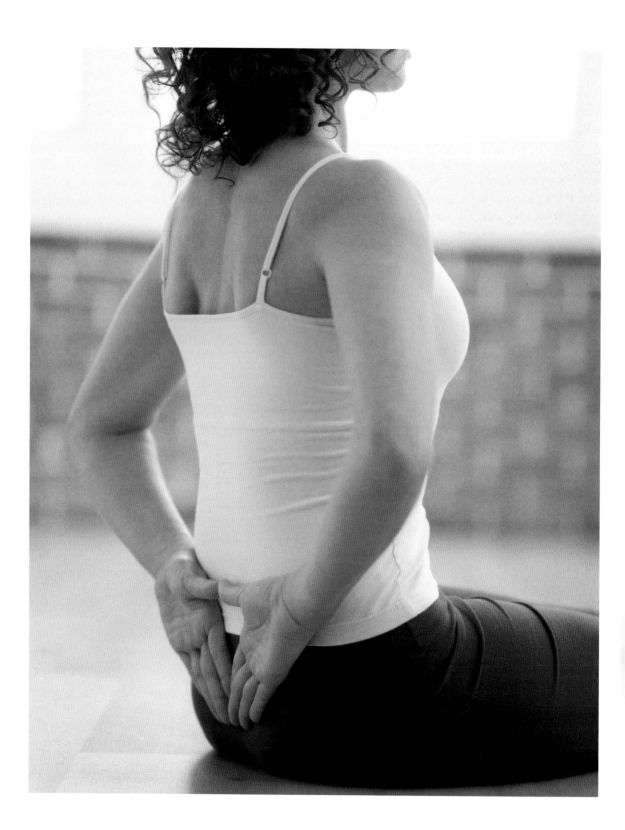

135 Tighten and Tone for Strong Abs

If your abs are feeling a little soft, try this series of abdominal-strengthening yoga poses, which lets you gradually increase the intensity of your workout as you gain muscle tone.

Throughout these poses, use the Diamond Base position (pictured at left) to keep your back supported. Place your hands against your lower back, palms out, with the tips of your thumbs and index fingers touching. Remember to also press your lower back down firmly. If your back lifts up—a sign that you're straining it—stop and rest.

1 Lie on your back and place your left foot on the floor so your bent left knee points upward. Keeping your right leg straight and your foot flexed, inhale as you lift your leg as high as is comfortable (no more than 90 degrees). As you exhale, lower your leg, keeping your foot flexed. Do this six times, then repeat with your other leg.

2 To make this basic lift a little more challenging, keep your resting leg straight along the floor as you work the other leg. Alternate legs, lifting each leg six times. Remember to build intensity gradually; if you feel any strain, go back to the easier version.

3 When you're ready, you can increase your workout by holding your resting leg straight up toward the ceiling while you lift and lower the other leg. Work each leg six times.

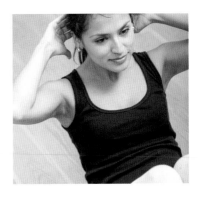

Work Abs for Back Health

A desire for washboard abs might motivate you to work those core muscles, but having strong abdominals also helps prevent lower-back pain, a potentially debilitating affliction that affects four out of five Americans at some point in their lives.

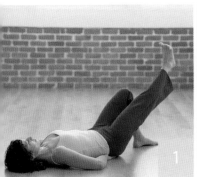
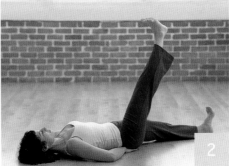
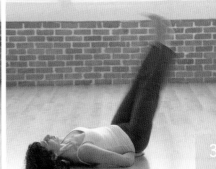

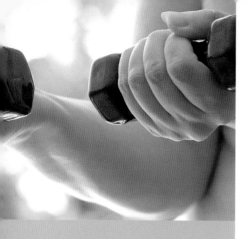

136

Maximize Your Weight Routine

Incorporating free weights into your exercise routine is key to maximizing your results. To make sure that you don't strain your wrists and arm muscles, start with weights that feel good in your hands, ergonomically speaking. They should seem fairly light at first but should challenge you as you perform a number of repetitions. As you gain strength, move on to a heavier set of weights (for example, from three pounds to five and then to eight). The last three repetitions should always feel a bit challenging but not so difficult that you can't maintain good form.

137 Get Results with Basic Arm Moves

Arm muscles are among the most obliging in the body, responding quickly to exercise. Just perform these moves every other day for a few weeks and you'll see the difference.

1 Stand tall, holding a weight in your left hand. Step forward with your right leg; bend your right knee and position it in line with your second toe. Rest your right hand on your thigh, just above your bent right knee. Keep left leg comfortably in back of you, with your toes facing straight ahead and your knee slightly bent. Draw in your ab muscles, as if you're pulling your navel toward your spine. Keep your shoulders and hips square, angle your tailbone slightly up, and make sure your neck is straight as you gaze at the floor. Lift your left upper arm in line with your torso, bending your elbow about 90 degrees.

2 With your upper body and legs as still as possible, on the exhale, straighten your arm, pivoting from the elbow. Keep your wrist straight and upper arm stable and along the same line as your torso. Bend your arm to return to the starting position. Repeat 15 times. To help you establish the correct rhythm, raise your arm up for two counts, hold for one, and slowly lower down for four counts. Then, holding the weight in your right hand and bending your left leg forward, repeat this exercise 15 times with your right hand.

3 Now, holding a weight in each hand, stand up straight with your feet hip-width apart and your arms resting at your sides. Your toes should be pointed straight ahead, your shoulders down and back, and your knees slightly bent. Draw in your abs and look straight ahead.

4 On the exhale, raise both of your arms, thumbs up, at a 30-degree angle out from your body until your hands reach eye level. Keep your shoulder blades down and collarbones wide, and don't let your back arch. Hold for one count and then, on the inhale, return your arms slowly to the starting position. Repeat this step 10 times.

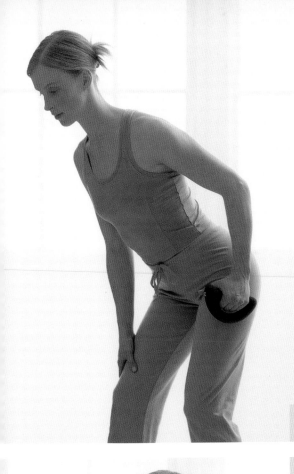
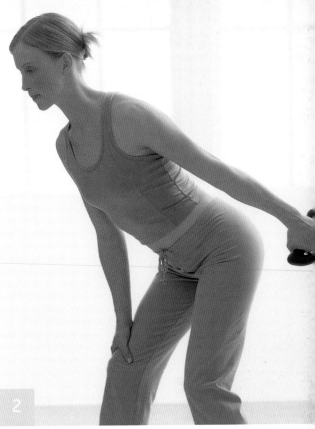

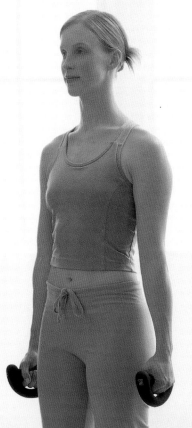
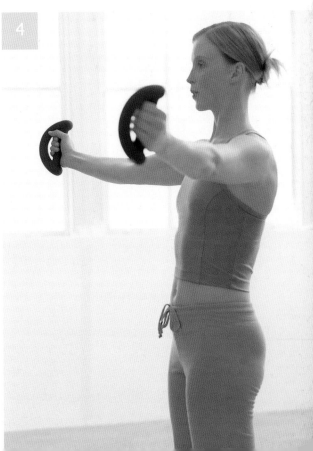

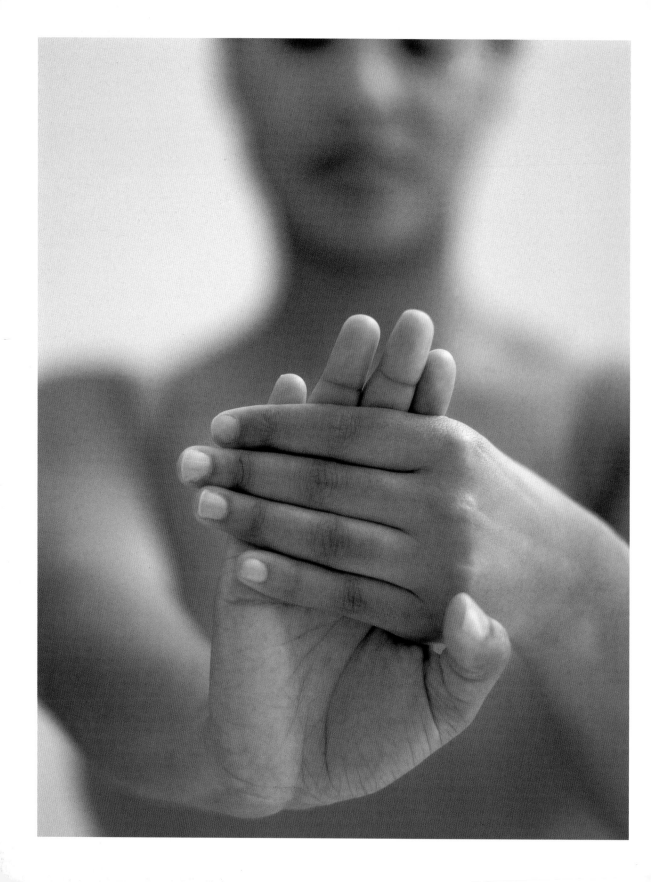

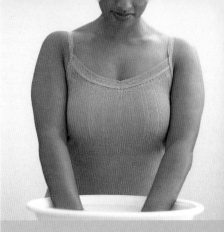

138 Try Wrist-Friendly Stretches

Protect your hands and wrists with a do-anywhere exercise to help prevent repetitive-motion problems. Stretching your wrist and hand muscles can help make them more resistant to injury.

1 Sit in a chair and extend your right arm out in front of you with your palm facing out and your fingers pointing upward, or rest your right elbow comfortably on a table, a desktop, or the arm of a chair.

2 Place the fingers of your left hand horizontally across the fingers of your right hand (see photo at left) and push the heel of your right hand outward as you gently pull toward you with your left hand just to the point of resistance. Breathe deeply. (Note: If you're not resting your right elbow on a hard surface, be sure to keep it slightly bent.)

3 Hold for 30 seconds. Focus on letting go when exhaling.

4 Repeat the move on your other hand. Stretch only to what feels comfortable; you should feel a bit of a stretch, but don't push too hard, and stop at any sign of pain.

139 Soak Away Wrist Tension

If you're suffering from the effects of a repetitive-stress injury, try a ten-minute witch hazel soak to relieve some of the discomfort.

1 Fill a large bowl with hot water and add a half cup of witch hazel. Submerge your hands and wrists. For the first five minutes, keep your hands still in any position that feels comfortable.

2 For the next couple of minutes, keep your hands submerged as you alternate between making fists and spreading your fingers wide.

3 End by circling your wrists slowly as if you are drawing a spiral in a clockwise direction, then move them counterclockwise.

140 Heal with Witch Hazel

Witch hazel has astringent and anti-inflammatory properties. Use it to soothe sore muscles, alleviate the itch of insect bites, and relieve the discomfort of hemorrhoids.

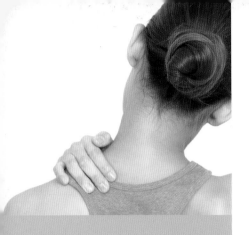

141

Release Muscle Fibers

Skeletal muscle fibers run parallel to one another, sliding against each other thousands of times a day as they relax and contract with every movement. Stress, poor diet, insufficient fluids, bad posture, fatigue, overuse, and other factors can cause these fibers to stick together, making you feel stiff and sore in places. Roll your thumb, fingers, knuckles, or elbows across the grain of the muscles to start to separate the stuck fibers, releasing the chemical glue binding them.

142 Ease Arm Muscles with Self-Massage

To warm up your arms before a workout or soothe joint or muscle pain afterward, try this self-massage, which combines compression, cross-fiber friction, and direct pressure.

1 With one hand braced on the back of your head, sink your fingertips into the front edge of your armpit to position them under your chest muscles. Squeeze your thumb and fingers together. Work the length of the muscle from top to bottom, squeezing and rolling across the ropy muscle fibers. Repeat three times (or until you feel the muscles relax), and then work on the other arm.

2 Increase circulation and release the tension in your biceps with compression. Rest your elbow on your knee or on a table. With your palm flat against the inside of your biceps just above your elbow and your fingers wrapped around your arm, squeeze firmly, then release. Rhythmically pump in this manner as you move from elbow to shoulder. Do three times; then repeat on the other arm.

3 To help relieve tension in your forearm, sink the fingers of one hand into the muscles on the top of your opposite forearm and firmly rub across the muscles from side to side, feeling them roll under the pressure (this is what's known as cross-fiber friction). Work them for three to five seconds. Release your grip slightly and repeat the move as you make your way from elbow to wrist. When you've covered the length of your forearm, repeat on the other arm.

4 If any areas on your arms are sore, soothe them with direct pressure. Take a deep breath, and, as you exhale, press your thumb slowly into a sore spot. The pressure should be firm, but not enough to cause acute discomfort. Breathe normally and hold the point for 10 to 30 seconds before releasing the pressure gradually. Press, hold, and release three times on each sore spot.

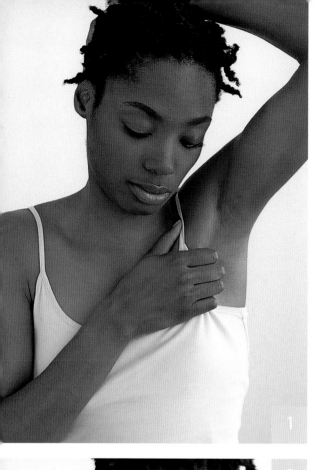

1

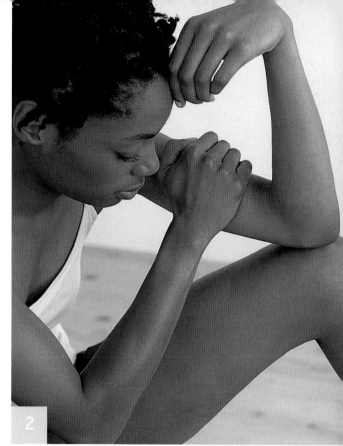

2

3

4

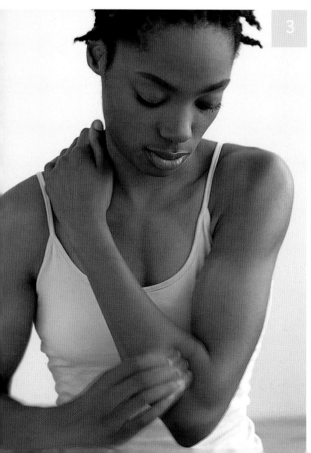

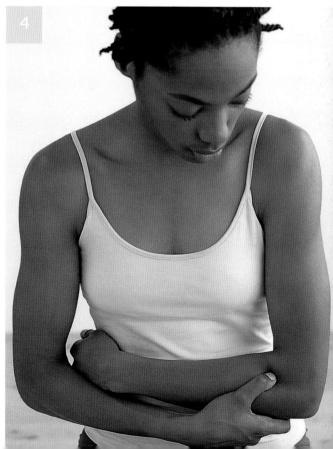

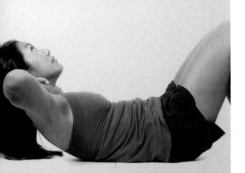

143

Don't Count on Spot Exercises

Think you can get rid of the fat on your thighs or tummy with spot exercises? Think again. Exercising or lifting weights will strengthen and tone muscles in those areas, but workouts alone won't make the fat go away. To get rid of subcutaneous layers of fat, you have to lose weight.

144 Get Great Legs with Simple Exercises

This exercise sequence works the glutes, hamstrings, quads, and lower legs, while honing your balance and weight-shifting skills, which are critical in skiing and other sports.

1 Stand up straight with your legs slightly wider than hip-width apart, hands at your sides. Tuck in your chin slightly and distribute your body weight evenly between the balls of your feet and heels; tighten your abdominals by drawing your belly button toward your spine.

2 On an inhale, squat: Drop your butt back and fold at the break of your legs. Lift your chest and extend your arms in front of you for balance. Bring your thighs as parallel to the floor as is comfortable, but do not strain. Aim your knees over the second toe of each foot.

3 Come out of the squat, pushing off from your heels as you exhale and lowering your arms as you rise. Once you are back up to a standing position, lift your right leg off the floor and extend it ten degrees behind your body while balancing on your left leg. Keep your spine lengthened and your abs tight; squeeze the right glute. Then bring the leg back to the floor and begin another squat; this time lift your left leg back. Alternate legs until you have completed ten repetitions on each leg, for a total of 20 squats.

145 Beat Age-Related Weight Gain

Women gain weight as they age. Women typically gain weight over time because their basal metabolic rate (BMR)—the number of calories burned in a day simply by being alive—drops as muscle mass naturally converts to fat. Since muscles burn eight times as many calories as fat, losing muscle mass reduces your BMR. To counter this process, create (or enhance) an aerobic exercise routine so that you'll burn more calories, and do strength training to keep your muscle-to-fat ratio up.

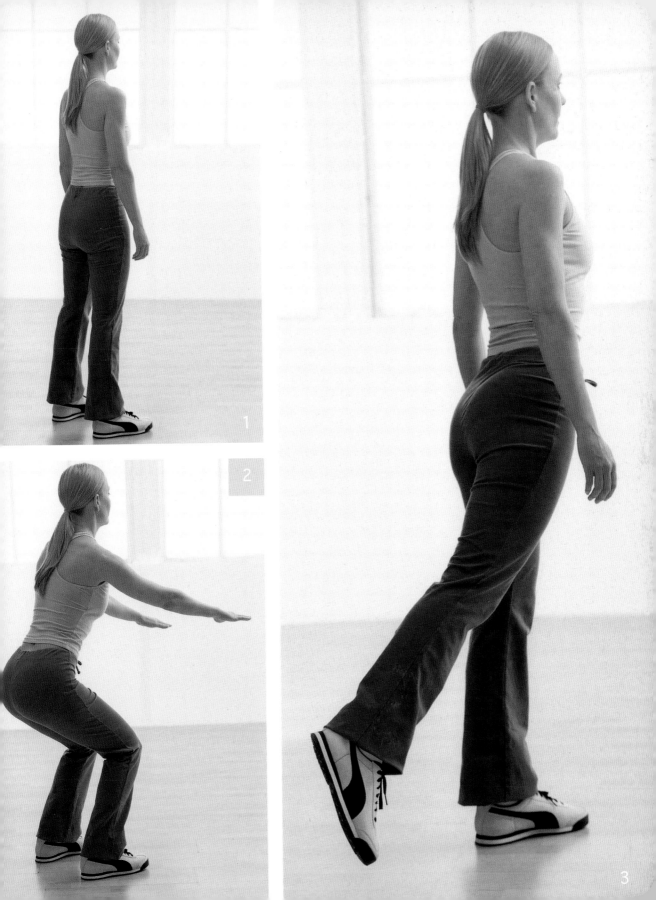

1

2

3

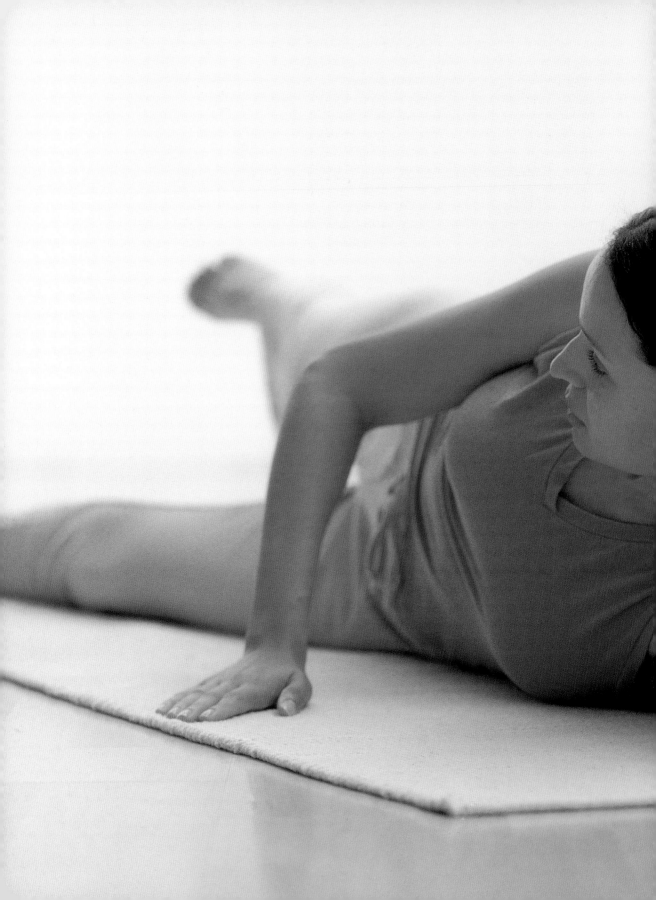

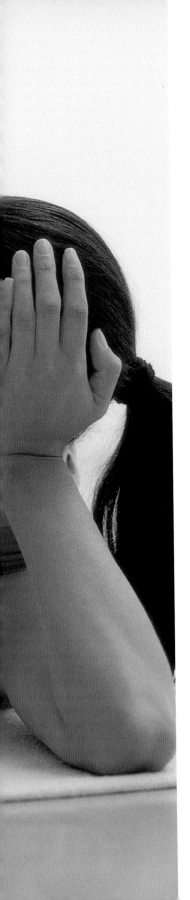

146 Work Your Powerhouse for a Strong Core

Pilates routines help tone muscles by focusing on lengthening and strengthening them, rather than using quick, abrupt contractions. The sequence of Pilates exercises on the following pages helps develop muscles in the abdomen, back, and hips—areas many women need to strengthen to develop better balance and greater flexibility. Also, synchronizing opposite arms and legs helps improve coordination.

When practicing Pilates, concentrate on the extension—as well as the contraction—in each movement to avoid arching your back, and be sure to keep your navel pulled back toward your spine as you work. Also, keep the abdominals active as you lie on your stomach to help prevent excessive compression of the lower back.

Why the emphasis on core muscles? Pilates exercises focus on the muscles that lie deep within the center of the body—muscles known as the "powerhouse" in Pilates circles—including the ab, back, thigh, and buttock muscles. Realigning, strengthening, and lengthening these core muscles improves posture, reduces the risk of injury, enables greater range of motion, and promotes flexibility.

147 Take a Lateral Approach to Breathing

Because we normally breathe using our diaphragm, which expands when we breathe in, it can take some time to adjust to the Pilates technique of lateral breathing. When performing Pilates exercises, contract your ab muscles; picture them supporting your torso like a corset. At the same time, inhale deeply and try to expand your rib cage to the sides and back. Continue to pull in your abs as you exhale completely. Inhalations and exhalations are often coordinated with specific movements in Pilates.

148 Target Core Muscles

This set of Pilates exercises will strengthen your abdomen, back, and hips. Practice these samll, focused movements at a slow pace to build core muscle and improve posture. Avoid exaggerating the positions in order to minimize injury.

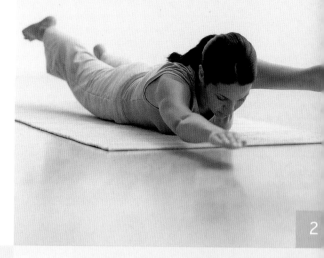

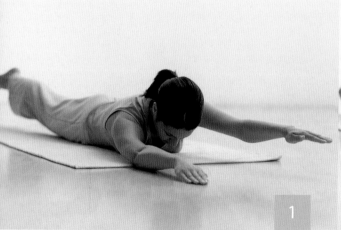

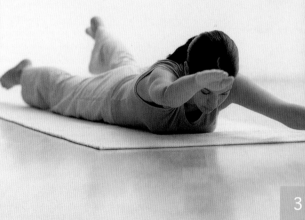

1 This exercise is called "swimming." Lie on your stomach, with your arms straight over your head, feet hip-width apart. Lift your head but look down; keep your neck and spine long, abs pulled in, and feet pointed. Inhale and lift up one arm and the opposite leg about eight inches. Stretch the raised limbs out, then exhale and lower them. Inhale and lift the opposite arm and leg, stretch the lifted limbs out, and then lower them. Alternate sides for two to three minutes.

2 To make this a more advanced exercise, lift both of your arms and legs off the ground. Alternate moving opposite arms and legs in a swimming motion.

3 As you get stronger at this exercise, speed up the swimming motion. If your back hurts or you are straining, go back to the simple, alternating swimming movement, with two limbs on the floor at all times.

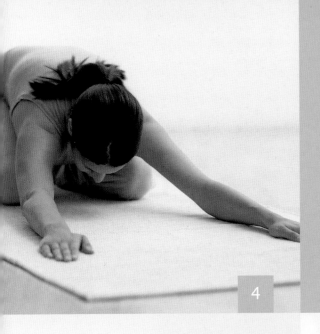

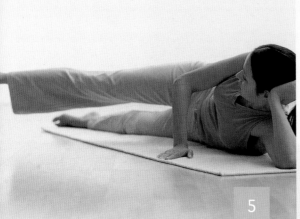

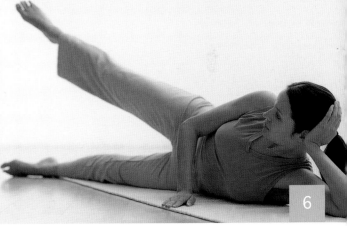

Classes that utilize traditional Pilates equipment are typically expensive private or semiprivate lessons. Fortunately, many Pilates exercises are designed to be performed on a mat. You can do mat exercises at a less-expensive group class or at home. This Pilates sequence is especially good for strengthening and stretching your back.

4 Relax your back by going into what's known as a prayer stretch: Sit back over your heels, with your knees slightly apart, your chest relaxed and close to the floor, and your arms stretched out comfortably in front. Hold for about 20 seconds, breathing deeply but naturally the whole time.

5 Lie on your side. Support your head with one arm; place the other in front of you. Lift the top leg a few inches and swing it forward with a flexed foot. Then swing the leg back about ten degrees; point your toes. Keep your torso still. Do eight times with each leg.

6 Lift your top leg up and down, with the leg slightly turned out and toes pointed. Repeat the leg lifts eight times on each side.

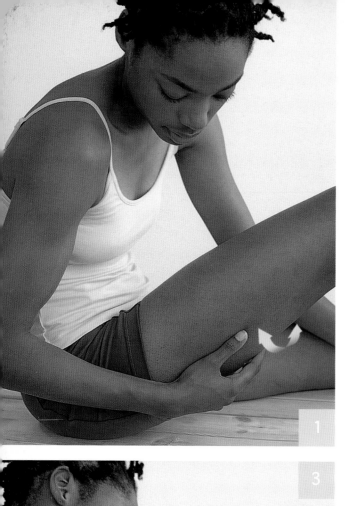

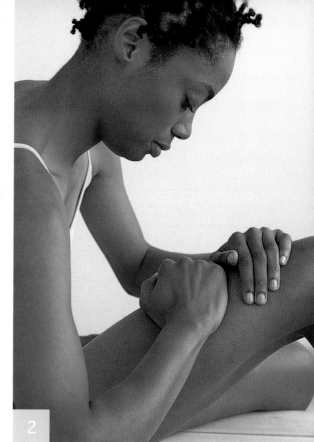

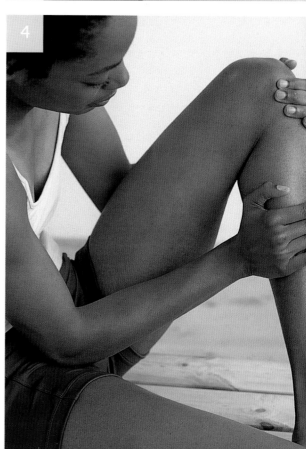

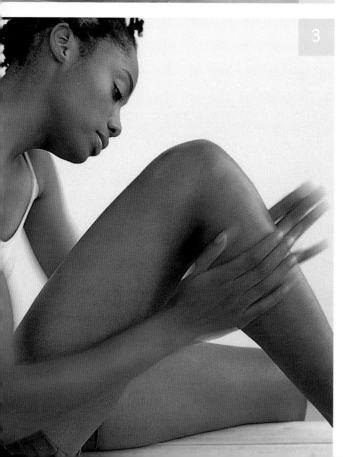

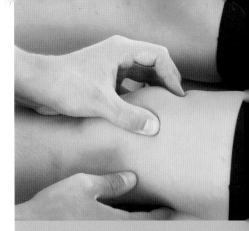

149 Love Your Legs with a Sports Massage

Just like stretching your legs, these easy self-massage techniques will help warm you up, pump you up, and even undo damage.

1 Relax tension in your hamstrings with a little jiggle before exercise. Sit on the ground or a bench, bend one knee up slightly, and grasp the muscles on the underside of that thigh with one hand. Begin waggling them loosely from side to side. Move up and down the length of your thigh, jostling your leg muscles as you go. Do six times on each leg.

2 Compress your quadriceps. Sit and bend one knee up slightly, as before. With the heels of both palms, press down into your thigh muscles, squeezing toward the bone in a pumping action. Release the pressure and move to a new spot, repeating from knee to hip. For extra power, rock your body forward as you press in, and lean back on your release. Work both of your legs from the knee to the hip six times.

3 Roll the calf muscles. With palms pressed into the fleshy part of your calf, rapidly push up with one hand while pulling down with the other, creating a rolling motion, for 30 seconds. Work both legs.

4 Starting near one ankle, press with the heel of your palm straight in toward the bone, and release. Pump the calf muscles in a rhythmic manner, moving toward your knee. Repeat this set of compressions three times, then work the other leg.

150 Soothe Minor Sports Injuries with PRICE

Most sports injuries are sprains (damage to ligaments, which link bones together), strains (damage to tendons, which bind muscles to bones), and contusions (bruises). A good strategy for treating minor injuries is PRICE: Protect (use bandages, elastic wraps, or splints, if needed), Rest (don't exercise the injured body part), Ice (10 to 15 minutes every hour for the first four hours, then four times a day for two to three days), Compress (with an elastic cloth bandage), and Elevate (use gravity to drain fluid away from injured tissue). After two to three days, switch to heat to relieve discomfort.

151

Keep It Short and Sweet

Invigorating sports massages can be beneficial either before or after a workout. They are usually short in duration; just a few minutes is restorative without being overly relaxing for the recipient. The brief rubdowns also give the hardworking massager a break, as they require quite a bit of energy to give.

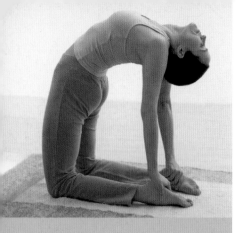

152

Strive, but Don't Strain

Yogis believe that it's important to balance *tapas* ("heat" in Sanskrit), the practice of asceticism and discipline for growth, and *ahimsa* ("non-harming"), the principle of caring for yourself and others. Too much *tapas* manifests itself in physical strain. When practicing yoga, strive for your maximum effort without strain.

153 Practice Yoga's Victory Breath

The Victory Breath is a classic yoga breathing technique that helps you gather steadiness and strength, a useful practice when you're trying to move into more challenging yoga poses. For these advanced yoga poses, such as the one pictured at right, use the Victory Breath to strengthen and stabilize both your mind and body.

Settle into a comfortable sitting position on the floor or on a rolled-up towel. Exhale slowly through your nose as you gently contract the top of your throat. This involves the same muscular movement in your throat as when you exhale through your mouth to fog up a mirror; you're just doing it with your mouth closed. (In yoga, breathing is almost always done with the mouth closed.) Inhale slowly and deeply, continuing to keep the throat slightly constricted. Listen for a faint hissing sound. (If your breath catches in your throat like a snore, you're contracting the throat too much.)

Use the focus required when practicing the Victory Breath to steady your mind and your body while entering into or holding any pose, particularly those you find challenging.

154 Avoid Competitive Yoga

In yoga class, especially if you're a beginner, be careful not to try to keep up with other students, who might be more advanced. How do you tell if you're pushing too hard? Signs of strain include trembling, ragged breathing or a tendency to hold your breath, dizziness, anxiety, and discomfort. Move slowly, gently, and with awareness of your own goals and limitations. Measure your ability by your own improvement, not by comparing yourself to the performance of others.

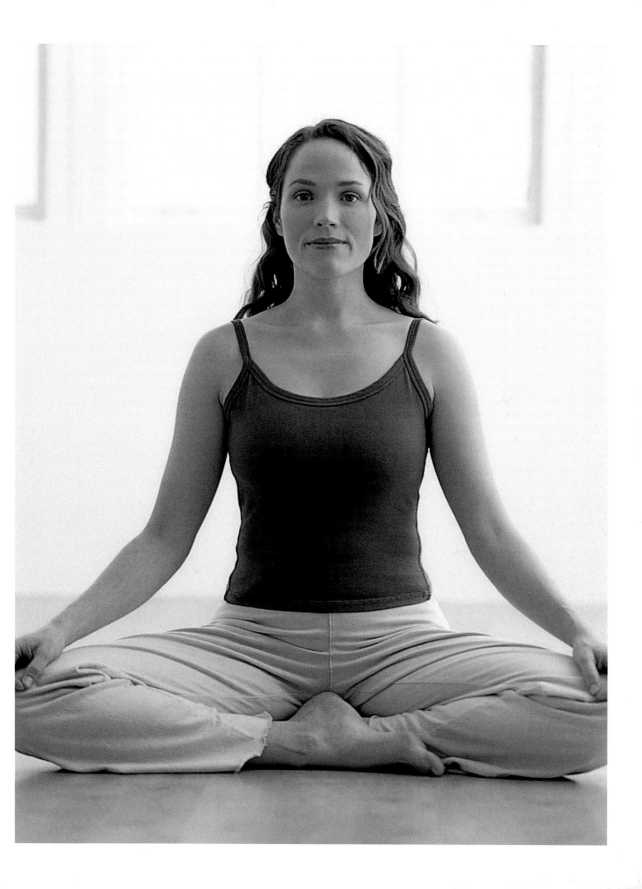

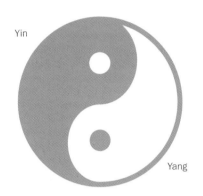

Yin

Yang

Decipher Yin and Yang

The yin–yang symbol depicts the principle at the heart of tai chi: the interplay between what seem to be opposing energies. The dark half of the circle represents yin (a passive, receptive, feminine, and still energy); the light half represents yang (an active, creative, masculine, and moving energy). Yield to the passive energy of yin when you inhale and feel the active energy of yang when you exhale. Yin and yang are complements, not opposites. The dot within each half of the circle symbolizes that the potential for yang is implicit in yin, and vice versa.

155 Benefit from Simple Weight Shifts

In this tai chi movement, called Brush Knee, the subtle force of shifting your weight helps you develop balance, agility, and strength. Work slowly to gain the maximum benefit.

1 Begin with your legs together and slightly bent. Your right foot should be in back of your left and the heel should be up; keep your left foot firmly planted on the floor. Raise your hands to chin level, with your fingers parted and facing outward. Your left hand should be close to your head; your right arm should be extended, with the elbow bent slightly. Look out over your right hand.

2 Step out with your right foot, keeping both feet flat. Tai chi instructors say that your left leg should feel "full" (that is, it should be bearing most of your weight); your right leg should feel "empty."

3 Lower your right arm, bending your elbow slightly and keeping your palm flat and facing the ground. Push out with your left hand, with your fingers pointing up. As always in tai chi, try to keep your joints—wrists, knees, elbows, and so on—relaxed, with soft angles, as you move. When you're done, you can repeat these steps on the other side, and then alternate both sides again.

156 Build Muscles, Tai Chi Style

Don't be deceived! The slow, flowing movements of tai chi might look as if they provide little challenge to muscles. But because you do the exercises in a crouching position and shift your balance from one leg to another, you strengthen your leg muscles, while avoiding the risks of high-impact exercise. The twisting and turning motions in tai chi also help develop your abdominal muscles. To get the most benefit, move slowly and mindfully through each sequence.

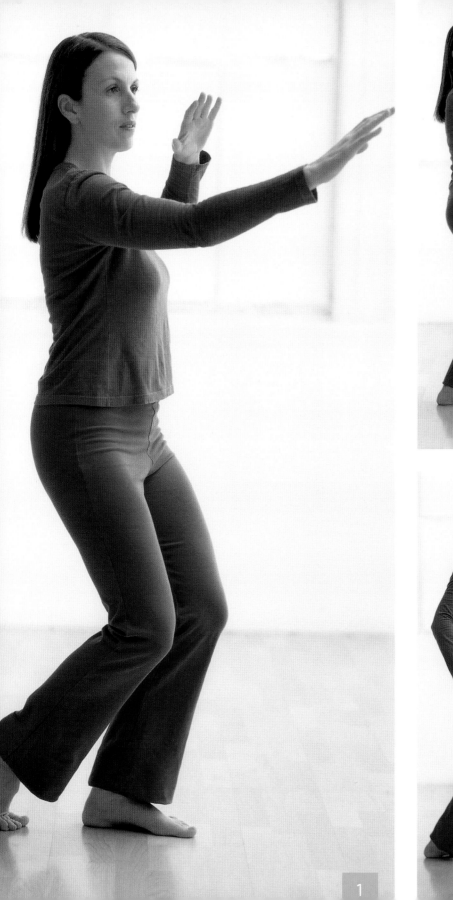
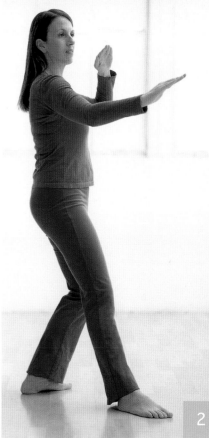
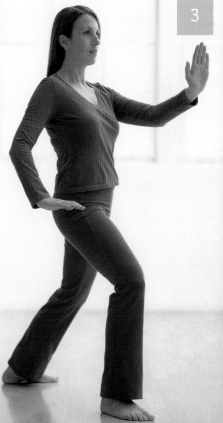

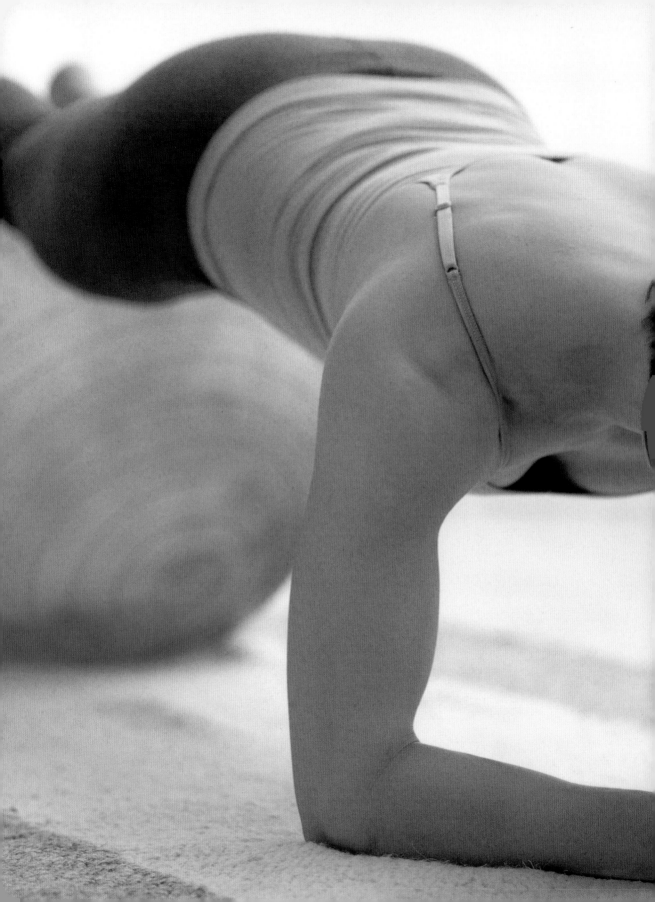

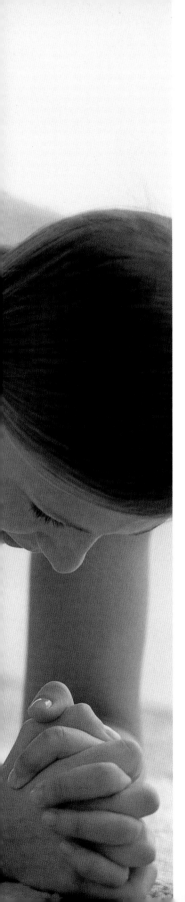

157 Build Balance and Strength on a Ball

A staple in Pilates exercises, the use of a large, inflatable ball can help develop muscles that don't normally get challenged even in the most rigorous sports or classes.

Rolling around on a large ball may seem like child's play. But done correctly, ball work can be incredibly challenging. Exercising on a ball helps you develop core muscles and a moment-to-moment balance that most floor exercises don't require. Using a ball also lets you do Pilates strengthening and stretching exercises that would otherwise require expensive equipment. Together, the ball and the Pilates tradition can help you align your body and strengthen your torso, both of which contribute to the long, lean physique that's characteristic of those who regularly practice Pilates.

You can buy a 55- to 65-centimeter fitness ball at almost any store that sells exercise equipment. (Generally people under five-foot-eight will be most comfortable with a 55-centimeter ball.) It helps to use the ball on a carpet—or, even better, a sticky yoga mat—so the ball doesn't slip around too much. Be sure to choose a real fitness ball as opposed to, say, a child's inflatable ball. Fitness balls are made to withstand more pressure and movement.

158 Stretch Your Back on the Ball

While a fitness ball is a very effective strength-building tool, you can also use it to stretch your back. Experiment by draping yourself, stomach or back down, on the ball, and positioning the ball so that your body feels supported and you feel a gentle stretch. Maintain each stretch for 30 seconds or longer. Stop if you feel any pain.

159 Find Balance on a Ball

In this Pilates workout, your muscles have to work harder to maintain your balance on the unstable surface of the ball. Body alignment is key; if you find yourself falling out of position, take a break until you can regain proper form.

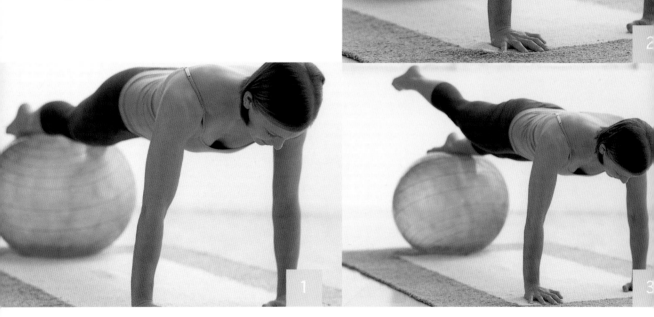

1 Balance in a push-up position with your arms on the floor, fingers pointing forward, and the tops of your feet on the ball. Push your shoulder blades away from your spine. Pull your ribs up, drawing in your ab muscles and tightening your buttocks. Don't arch your back or let your waist sag. Keep your neck straight and focus your eyes on the floor.

2 Lift one leg up, elongating your leg as much as possible and pointing your toes. Again, avoid arching your back or pushing your bottom up into the air. Maintain a level pelvis and draw your abs in.

3 Now work your other leg. Continue to alternate exercising your legs, lifting each one five to ten times. When you have finished, dismount carefully from the ball by bending your knees and bringing one leg down to the floor at a time.

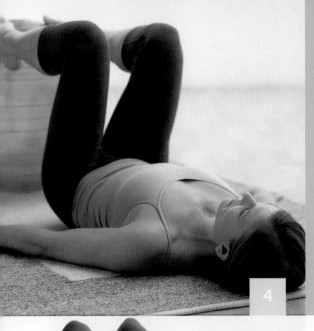

Step 1 in this sequence is a variation of the plank exercise, whereby you hold yourself up in a push-up position with your toes on the ground. This is also a yoga pose and a popular ab-strengthening exercise. Try doing this position with your feet on the ball, timing yourself every day at the same time. Stick with it and you will rapidly see your endurance and strength increase.

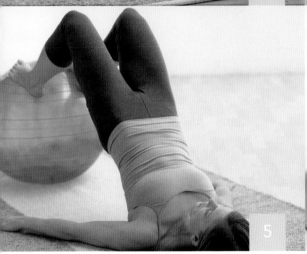

4 Lie on your back and put your feet on the ball so that your knees are at a 90-degree angle and your hands are out to your sides, palms down. Keep your abs pulled in, so your rib cage is pressed downward, toward the floor.

5 Push up on the ball with the bottoms of your feet, bend your knees, and rest on your shoulder blades. Avoid rolling onto your neck.

6 Pushing the ball away from you, extend your knees so that your body forms a straight line. Rest your heels on the ball, and try to keep your hips up. Draw the ball toward you. Pressing down with the soles of your feet, lower your pelvis to the floor. Repeat Steps 4 through 6 eight times.

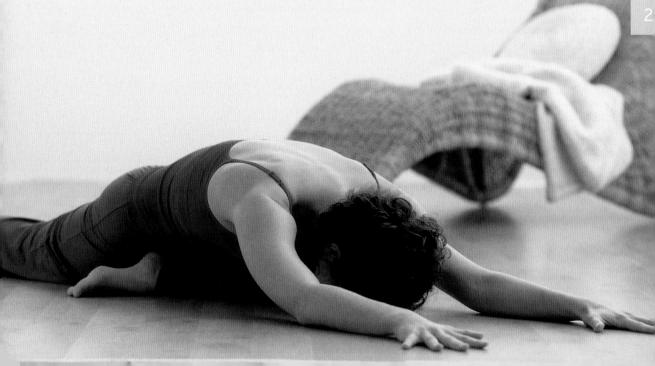

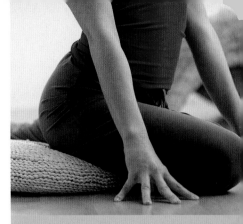

160 Try Variations on Pigeon Pose

Keep your yoga routine fresh and your body and mind stimulated by expanding your repertoire. Various Pigeon poses let you work with challenging but gratifying hip releases.

1 To perform Pigeon pose, get on all fours. Bring your left knee forward between your hands, with your foot positioned to the right so your leg forms an inverted V shape. Extend your right leg straight back and allow your hips to sink, keeping them level to the floor. Be careful not to roll onto your left thigh or strain your knees. Elongate your spine, lift your chest, and keep your palms on the floor and your shoulders loose and low. Hold for four to six breaths (but release at the first sign of any strain). To release, push down with your palms, lift your hips, and slide your left leg back. Repeat on the other side.

2 In Low Pigeon pose, your weight falls more on your arms and a bit less on your hips. From Pigeon pose, place your forearms on the floor shoulder-width apart. Lower your weight onto your forearms, relaxing over your bent leg. If this is comfortable, release more weight onto your bent leg by extending your arms completely and letting your head rest on (or hang toward) the floor. Note any resistance in your body, and encourage these muscles to surrender to the pose. Hold for four to six breaths. Release and repeat on the other side.

161 Protect Your Knees in Pigeon Pose

The variations of Pigeon pose provide challenging opportunities to work on releasing your hips. Your hips work in harmony with your knees, which may try to compensate for restrictions in the range of motion of your hip joints. When working to open your hip joints, take care not to strain your knees. Use a blanket to support your hips (see photo at right) if needed, and release the pose at any sign of strain. Remember, the yoga practice doesn't end when you leave your mat; observe how your body is affected by your practice immediately afterward and, as you practice regularly, over time.

162 Support Your Hips

If you find it difficult to keep your hips level in either Pigeon pose, try placing a firm pillow or a folded blanket under the hip of your bent-leg side. The farther your hips are from the floor, of course, the thicker the pillow or blanket needs to be. With practice, you gradually will need less support.

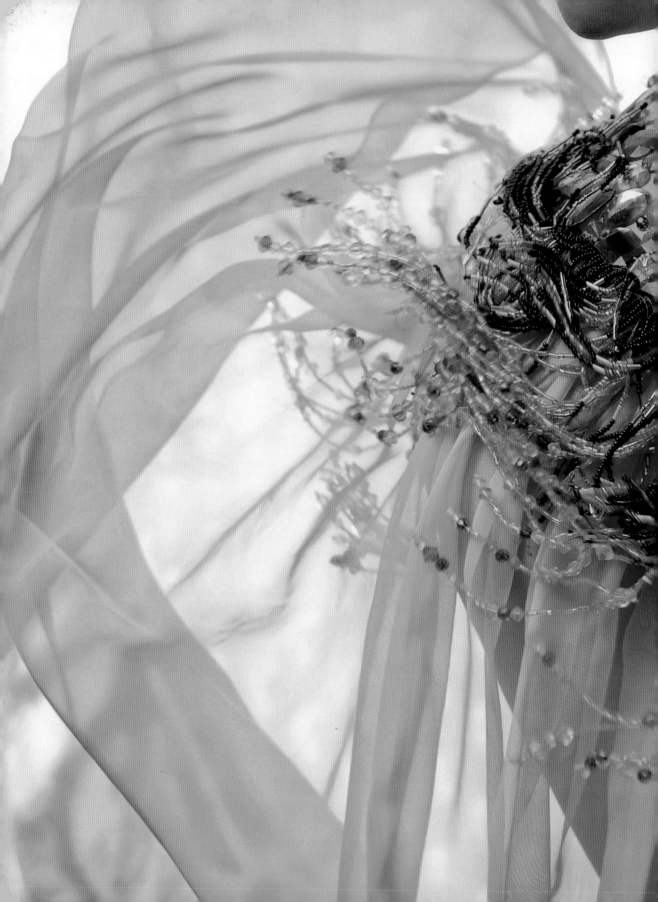

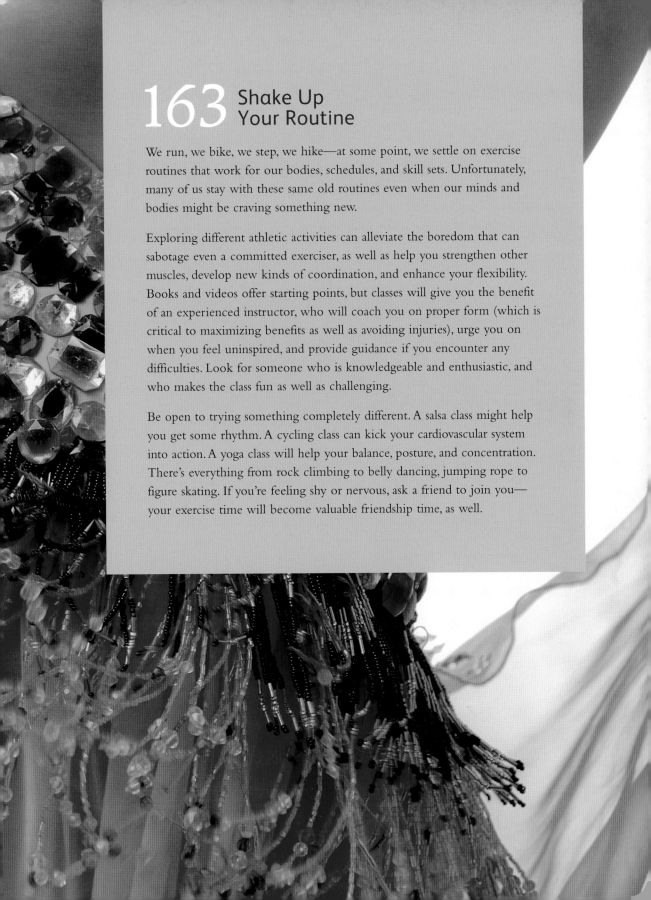

163 Shake Up Your Routine

We run, we bike, we step, we hike—at some point, we settle on exercise routines that work for our bodies, schedules, and skill sets. Unfortunately, many of us stay with these same old routines even when our minds and bodies might be craving something new.

Exploring different athletic activities can alleviate the boredom that can sabotage even a committed exerciser, as well as help you strengthen other muscles, develop new kinds of coordination, and enhance your flexibility. Books and videos offer starting points, but classes will give you the benefit of an experienced instructor, who will coach you on proper form (which is critical to maximizing benefits as well as avoiding injuries), urge you on when you feel uninspired, and provide guidance if you encounter any difficulties. Look for someone who is knowledgeable and enthusiastic, and who makes the class fun as well as challenging.

Be open to trying something completely different. A salsa class might help you get some rhythm. A cycling class can kick your cardiovascular system into action. A yoga class will help your balance, posture, and concentration. There's everything from rock climbing to belly dancing, jumping rope to figure skating. If you're feeling shy or nervous, ask a friend to join you—your exercise time will become valuable friendship time, as well.

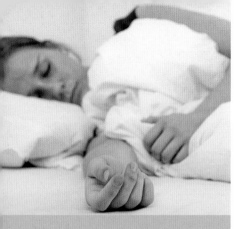

164
Baby Your Back

Back pain occurs all too easily among women, but it's also easy to develop good habits that will help ward it off. For instance, take frequent breaks to stretch when you work at a desk or a computer. Here are more tips to help your back.

- Sleep on your side, with a pillow that supports your neck. Avoid sleeping on your stomach.

- Don't lean into a mirror when grooming.

- Keep your purse, which causes your weight to shift to one side, light.

- Avoid high heels. Look for shoes with arch supports.

- Use a chair that best fits your size, preferably with an adjustable height.

165 Stretch Your Back with Cat and Cow

These satisfying yoga poses were inspired by the arc of a cat's back and a cow's swaybacked posture. Easy to do, they're great for stretching your back and strengthening core muscles.

1 For Cow pose, begin on all fours with your elbows straight but somewhat relaxed. Position your palms directly beneath your shoulders and your knees beneath your hips. (If you have weak or tender wrists, relieve the pressure on them by making fists, thumbs forward, with your hands on the floor.) Inhaling, press your belly down as your chest expands and gently lift your head and tailbone, lending a slight curve to your back, a bit reminiscent of a cow's swaybacked appearance.

2 Next, for Cat pose, exhale while contracting your diaphragm and abdomen, and lift your back as you lower your head and tailbone, like a cat engaged in a luxurious stretch.

Repeat the sequence for four to ten breaths. You might want to practice *mantra japa,* the repetition of a word or phrase. Done either silently or out loud and linked to coincide with the pace of your breathing, it can help you create a more meditative experience as you perform the poses. You may use any uplifting word or phrase. If none comes immediately to mind, try using the simple yet profound *shanti* (pronounced SHAHN-tee), which means "peace" in Sanskrit.

166 Learn to Lift Smarter

Many people lift heavy objects incorrectly, which is one of the most common causes of back injury. When picking up a heavy object, be sure to squat down, tuck in your buttocks, and hold the object close to you. Keep your back straight, and rise using the muscles of your legs to power the lift—not your vulnerable back.

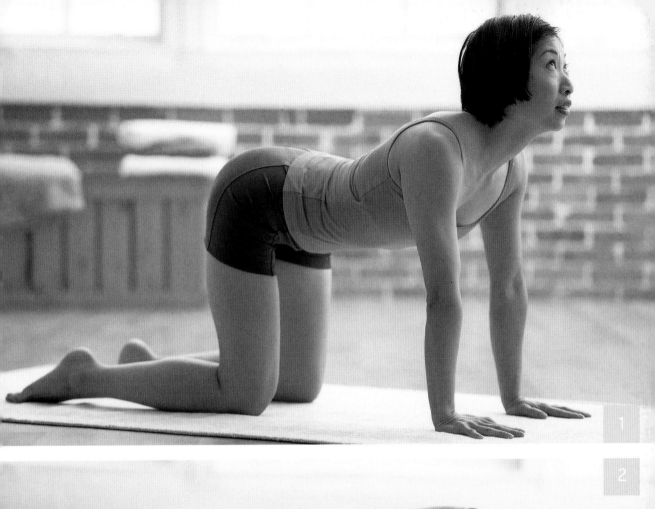

1

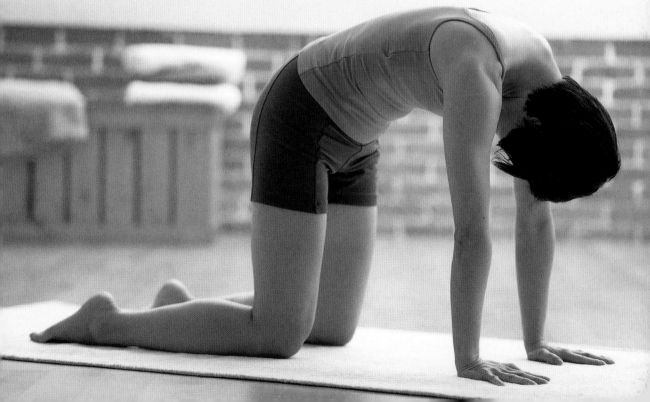

2

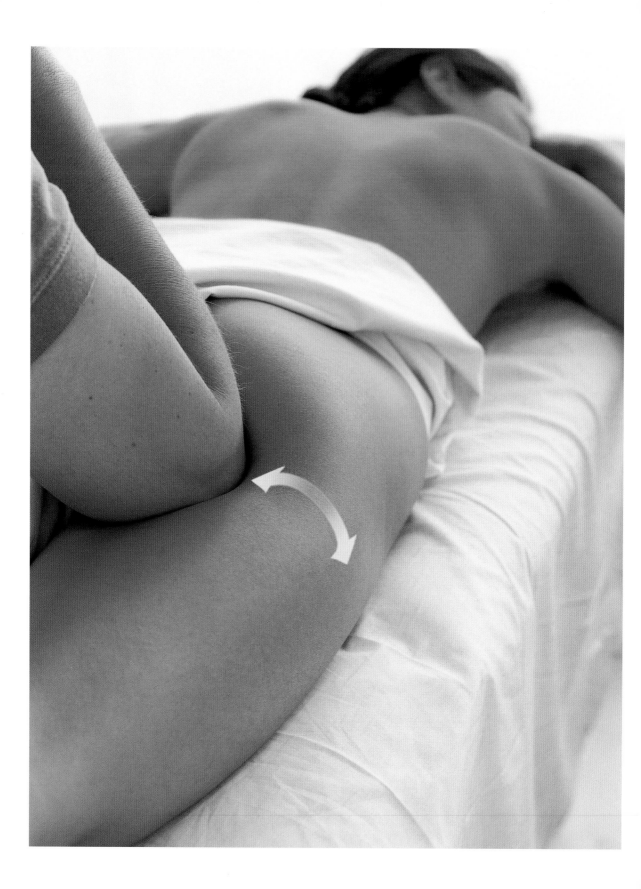

167 Loosen Tight Glutes with Massage

Trading glute massages with a friend will release pent-up tension. Here are the steps for your massage partner to follow:

1 To begin, position one of your elbows at the bottom of one of her gluteal muscles. Using firm pressure, glide up alongside her tailbone to the thick muscles of the glutes.

2 Then zigzag slowly back and forth across the muscles, working from the edge of the tailbone out to the wide part of the outer thigh and back in again. You'll know you're doing your job when you feel the fibers starting to separate.

3 Now position yourself to one side of your friend and press your fingertips into the far side of her opposite gluteal muscle. Leaning back, pull toward the tailbone with alternating hands. Do this ten times, then repeat the strokes on the other side.

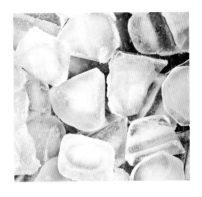

Recover After a Massage

Always drink plenty of water after receiving a cross-fiber massage. And if an area of your body is very sore, ice it for ten minutes after the massage.

168 Perform Careful Cross-Fiber Massage

Giving a cross-fiber massage can feel as if you are popping across taut ropes, but don't worry—this will help relax and soften the fibers. Soreness is common during and after cross-fiber work, but be careful not to overdo it. Excessive friction can injure the tissue. The rule of thumb: The deeper you go, the slower you go. Massage the muscles this way for about two or three minutes.

169 Partner Up for Double Boat Pose

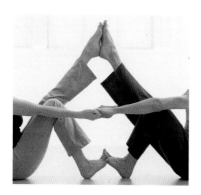

Steady as She Goes

The trick to getting into or out of Double Boat pose is to concentrate on one side at a time (don't try to lift both sets of legs simultaneously). As with any partner pose, you must remain sensitive to each other's pace, position, and level of comfort.

Feelings of connectedness, trust, and mutual support, plus a glorious stretch—all are benefits of Double Boat pose, a partner yoga pose that forms a striking silhouette. It is a double form of Boat pose, which earned its name for its resemblance to a sailing ship.

When done alone, Boat pose is an extremely demanding pose that requires strong abdominal muscles. Double Boat is a bit easier because you can use your partner to help brace your limbs and balance. A physical connection with your partner also helps strengthen your emotional connection, as you depend upon each other for support and can enjoy the meditative aspects of yoga together.

To start, sit on the floor face-to-face with your partner. Bend your knees and put your feet flat on the floor, with the toes touching. Clasp each other's hands (or forearms, if that's more comfortable), then slowly lift and straighten your legs, one side at a time, letting the soles of your feet touch the soles of your partner's feet. Keep your back straight rather than rounding it. As you each balance on your buttocks, lift in and up from your lower back, look at each other, and breathe slowly and deeply. Hold this pose for at least 20 seconds, and, eventually, try to extend it to one minute.

170 Grow Closer Through Yoga

The Sanskrit word *yoga* means "union." Although usually applied to achieving harmony between one's own mind and body, the concept of yoga can also be applied to two individuals—friends, family, romantic partners—coming together as one. Poses such as Double Boat allow two people to share their passion for yoga and feelings for each other. Even two people of dramatically different heights and weights can balance and support each other.

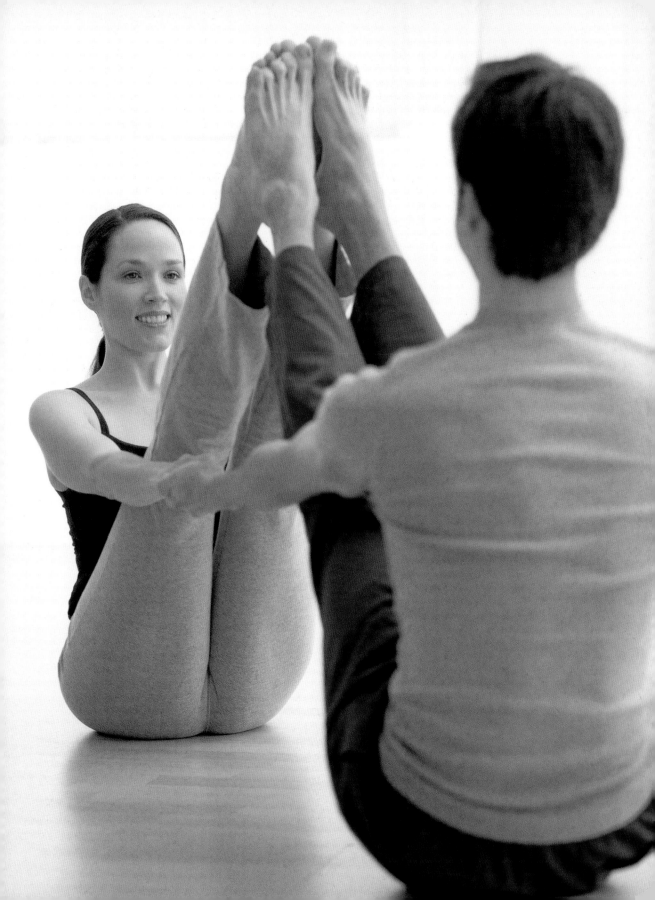

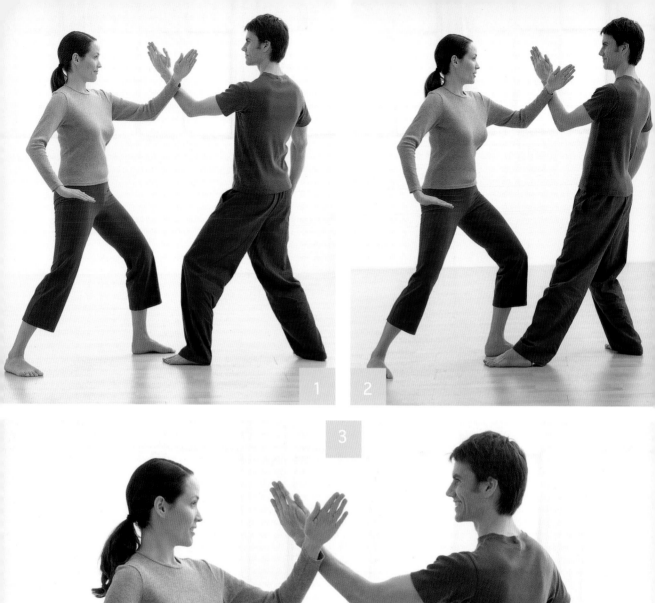

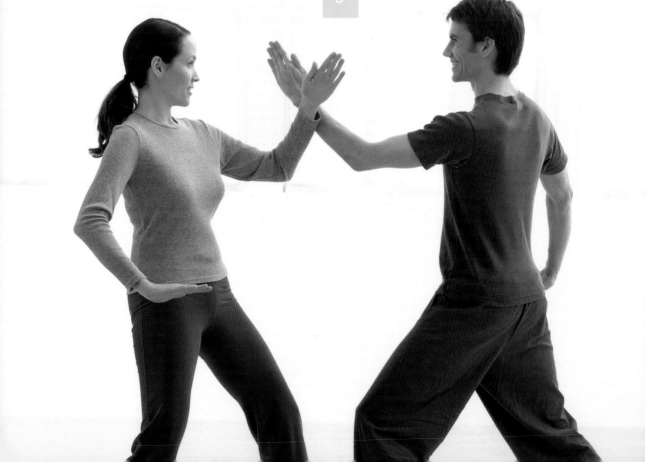

171 Increase Awareness of Each Other's Movements

Often used as sparring practice in the martial arts, Push Hands can be a shared tai chi exercise that helps you develop greater sensitivity to your partner's movements.

1 Starting an arm's distance away from your partner, step into the bow position: one leg forward and bent at the knee and one leg extended back. You both should have the same leg (that is, the right or the left) forward and feel balanced. Keep your head up and your tailbone down, so your spine is lengthened.

Each of you then raises the forward arm (the arm on the same side as your forward foot) to chest height, with the elbow softly bent. Keep the palm facing away from your partner's hand and your fingers straight. Rest the back of your forearm on the back of your partner's forearm, a bit like crossed swords. Hold your other hand down and at your side, with the elbow softly bent and your fingers out straight, palm facing the ground. Keep your shoulders down and relaxed.

2 Keeping your feet stationary, shift your weight forward as you gently push on your partner's forearm with your forearm. Your partner should yield to your force and shift his weight backward.

3 Next it's your partner's turn to press forward, shifting his weight toward you and exerting pressure with his forearm. This time, you respond by yielding and shifting your weight backward. Take turns with your partner—alternating pressing forward and yielding—with your feet remaining in place as your arms move back and forth in a tight, circular manner (picture the action of the wheels of a locomotive). Keep your hips loose so they can rotate freely, and absorb your partner's movements by keeping your knees bent, not by leaning back or tipping forward dramatically. Push hands in this manner for as long as you can both can stay relaxed and focused, alternating sides from time to time.

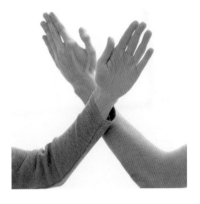

Armed and Ready

As you rock back and forth in Push Hands (Step 3), your forward hands and forearms can remain in the same position relative to each other. Or, if it feels more natural, they can travel up and down each other's arms, but not past the wrist or elbow.

indulge

Part of being a grown-up is knowing what you enjoy—the food you savor, the company you keep, and the activities you love. Sometimes, you might feel a little guilty about indulging in life's pleasures. But there's a time and a place for everything, and when it's your turn to revel in a little well-deserved pampering, we've got some ideas for you.

The activities in this chapter delight the senses—from perfuming your bedroom to exchanging massages by a flickering fire. These treatments go beyond simple maintenance to sensual joys. You'll find suggestions for revitalizing a tired body, reconnecting with your surroundings, and surrendering to a grown-up time-out. Whatever activity you choose, an indulgence should please the senses, calm the mind, and lift the spirit. And above all, it should make you happy. ✆

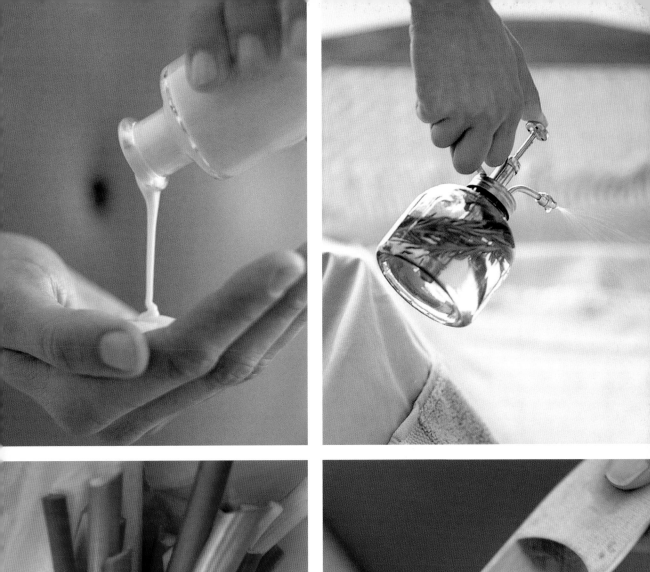
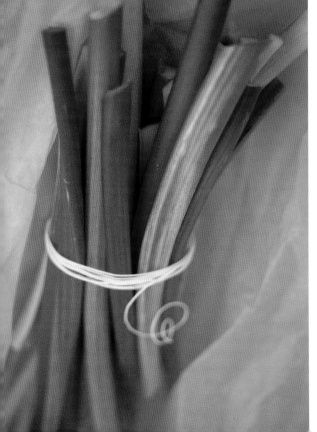
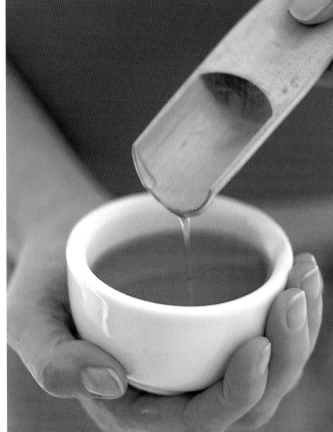

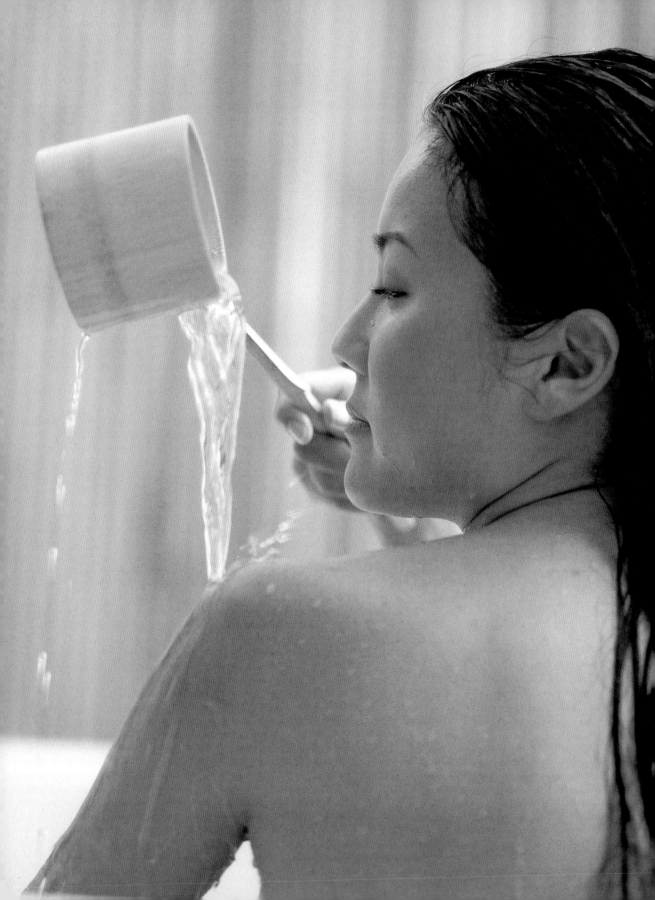

172 Enjoy Bath Therapy

When it comes to providing a respite from everyday cares, few things are more satisfying than a bath, especially when you use a ladle to caress your body with fragrant water.

1 Draw a very warm bath—not scalding, mind you, but hot enough that you will have to ease yourself into the water slowly. After the tub fills, add a blend of essential oils specially chosen for their comforting qualities (see the recipe at right, which will also help moisturize your skin). Before you enter the tub, stir the water with your hands to thoroughly mix the essential oils.

2 Get into the tub, and spend a few minutes just soaking in the warm water. Close your eyes and take deep, cleansing breaths.

3 Then, using a ladle, pour warm bathwater over your shoulders and the middle of your back. Notice and savor how the water soothes your muscles and helps calm your mind. Slowly ladle water onto the top and back of your head, being careful not to let it run over your face (essential oils can sting if they get in your eyes). Continue ladling bathwater onto the tops of your arms.

4 Keep ladling slowly and methodically as a form of meditation, visualizing the water washing away your worries.

5 When you've finished, lie back, close your eyes, and soak for another ten minutes or so, remaining in a peaceful, meditative state.

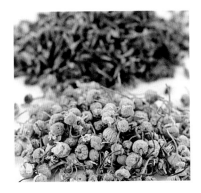

Comforting Bath Blend

1 teaspoon sweet almond oil
3 drops chamomile essential oil
3 drops lavender essential oil
2 drops geranium essential oil

173 Calm Down with Chamomile

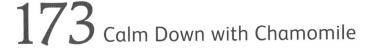

When drunk as tea, chamomile (either the Roman or German type) is said to relax the body and induce sleep; it also can help settle an upset stomach. As an essential oil, the herb (pictured) is often used to alleviate insomnia and nervousness. Chamomile's anti-inflammatory properties can also help soothe irritated or sunburned skin.

174 Set the Mood with Bedroom Aromatherapy

Using essential oils in the bedroom can conjure up associations of freshness, warmth, seduction, or peace—whatever mood you'd like your special refuge to reflect. As the room in which we sleep, dream, make love, and retreat, the bedroom deserves some extra attention and a dash of creativity. Decorating your bedroom to your liking and keeping it clean and free of clutter are crucial to making it feel like a calm place for retreat and indulgence. Helpful, too, is infusing your bedroom with just the right aroma.

Misting essential oils throughout your bedroom is a delightful way to create a mood. Just add a favorite essential oil or blend (see the recipe at left) to a spray-mister filled with distilled water. Besides spraying your mixture into the air, you can lightly spritz it on your bed linens, drapes, and carpet. Use light, clear oils to avoid stains, and don't spray over wood furniture. Choose a scent that suits your needs: Bergamot or Roman chamomile may help reduce stress levels. Lavender may help you relax. If romance is on your mind, ylang-ylang's exotic floral fragrance is believed to be an aphrodisiac, as are sandalwood and patchouli. Use lemon or grapefruit oils to freshen up the room; try eucalyptus to banish stale smells—and repel insects.

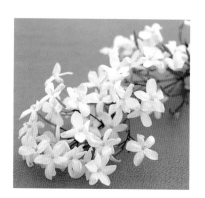

Indulgent Spray-Mist Blend

8 ounces distilled water
8 drops jasmine essential oil
7 drops lavender essential oil
7 drops sandalwood essential oil
3 drops vetiver essential oil

175 Set Your Bedroom Temperature Just Right

If you're having trouble sleeping, try turning down the thermostat. When you sleep your body temperature drops, and your body works to maintain that lower temperature. As a result, a bedroom that's too warm can interfere with sleep. The goal is to keep your bedroom on the cool side while still being comfortable, which is usually between 65 and 72 degrees Fahrenheit.

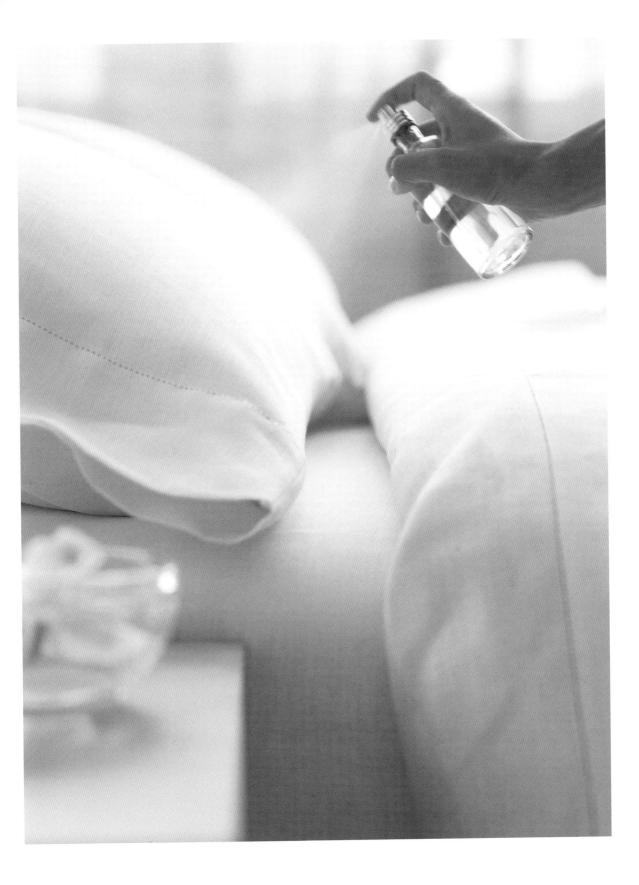

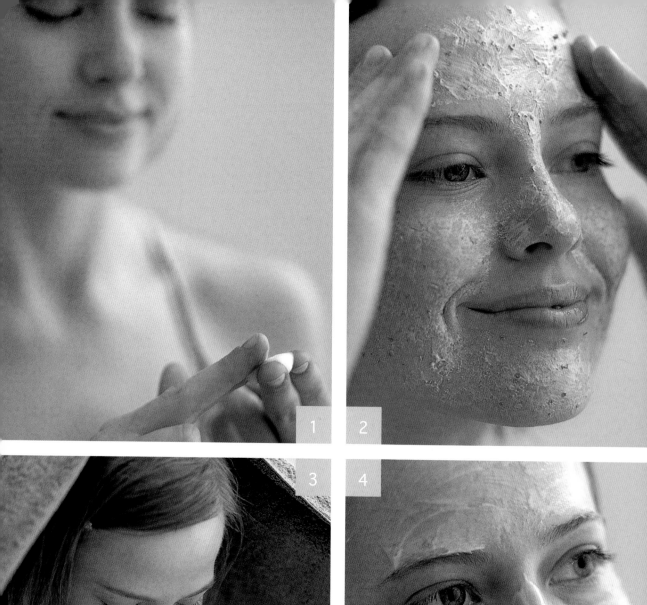

1

2

3

4

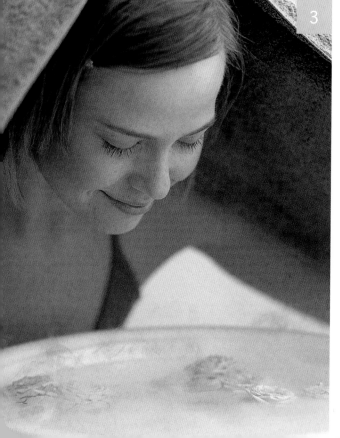

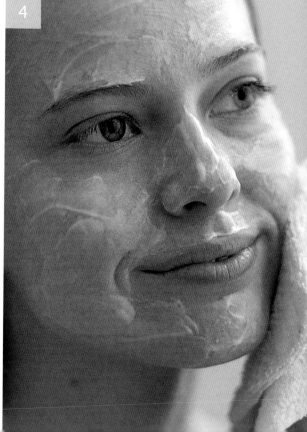

176 Glow with a Luxe Facial

Good daily care is essential to maintaining your skin's condition. For a luxurious experience, supplement your routine with a facial featuring an essential-oil steam that will enhance your healthy-looking glow.

1 Begin by cleansing your face with a product appropriate for your skin type. Wet your face, and apply a thumbnail-size dollop of cleanser, using gentle, circular motions to massage it over your entire face and neck. Rinse with tepid water and pat your face and neck dry.

2 Next, exfoliate your skin to remove dead cells, impurities, and oil. Exfoliating speeds up cell renewal and allows a smooth, glowing new layer of skin to emerge. Again, it's important to use a gentle product formulated for your particular skin type. Lightly rub your fingers in circles over your face, being careful to avoid the eye area. Rinse thoroughly with tepid water and pat dry.

3 Fill a bowl with boiling water. Add a few drops of essential oil: If your skin is dry, a rose-and-frankincense blend is an excellent choice. Lavender works well for dry-to-normal skin, chamomile helps soothe sensitive skin, and lemon suits oily skin. Mix the oil and water well. Lean over the bowl, keeping your face 10 to 12 inches away from the steaming water. Drape a bath towel over your head, creating a tent to trap the vapors. Steam your face for five to ten minutes.

4 While your skin is still damp from the steam, apply a facial mask formulated for your skin type and condition (for instance, a product that's moisturizing, purifying, or soothing). Spread a small amount over your face in a thin, even layer, and leave on for 10 to 20 minutes. Then use a wet cloth to remove the mask. Gently pat your face dry with a towel. Complete your luxurious facial by applying a moisturizing cream or serum compatible with your skin type.

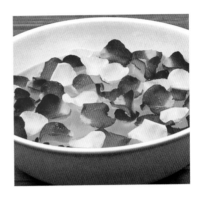

Be Ravishing with Rose Oil

Cooling, relaxing, and toning (but very pricey in undiluted form), rose essential oil is celebrated for its rejuvenating effects, especially for dry or mature skin. Rose oil is used frequently to soften wrinkles, moisturize, help reduce puffiness, and relieve clogged pores. In addition, its sweet floral aroma is quite soothing and helps promote restful sleep.

177 Turn Up the Heat with a Fireside Massage

Exchanging massages by firelight can be a relaxing, romantic, and wonderfully nonverbal way to connect with your partner. On a chilly evening, a fire's warmth is relaxing and comforting; the play of light and shadow is soothingly hypnotic. It is a perfect setting for practicing intimate touch. Snuggle up near the fireplace, and ask your partner to follow these instructions for a blissful massage. (If you're not too blissed out afterward, you might feel like reciprocating.)

1 Experiment with light, fast glides over the surface of her head, using gentle fingers to comb down through her hair. Begin the first strokes at the hairline on her forehead and sweep down to the ends. Then move back up to a different position at the hairline and repeat until you've gently stroked her entire head.

2 Sometimes the perfect touch for relaxation is a light sweep across the skin. Using the flat of your palms and easy pressure, place your hands low on your partner's back and sweep up to the base of her neck. Then fan your hands out to the edge of her shoulders and sweep back down the sides, returning to her waist and lower back. Repeat this pattern, encouraging your partner to breathe deeply and let the cares of the world slip away with each stroke.

3 To help work out the tension that tends to accumulate between the shoulder blades, stabilize your partner with one hand on a shoulder. With your other hand, press and run your thumb into the muscles between her shoulder blades and spine. Follow the edge of each shoulder blade from top to bottom, gliding up and down. Start with gentle pressure and work more deeply as the muscles relax.

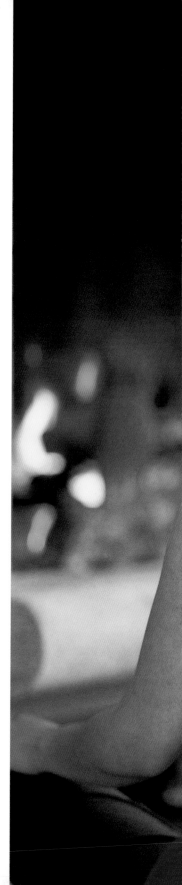

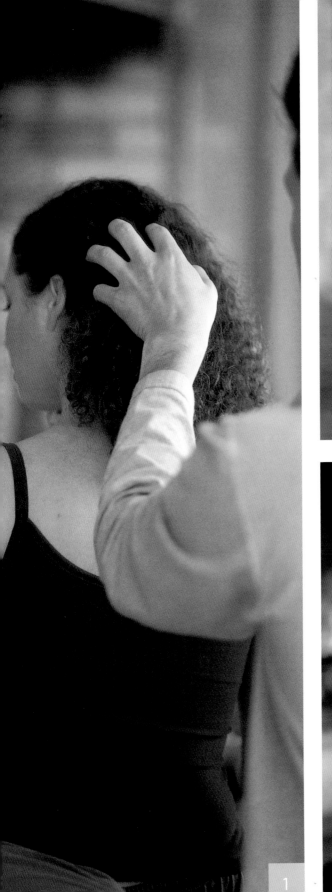

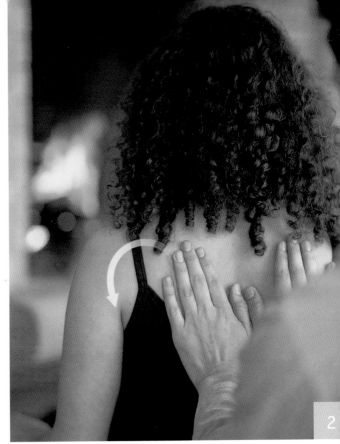

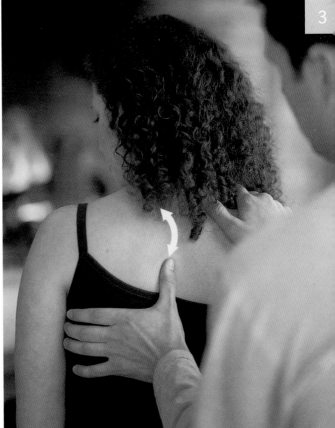

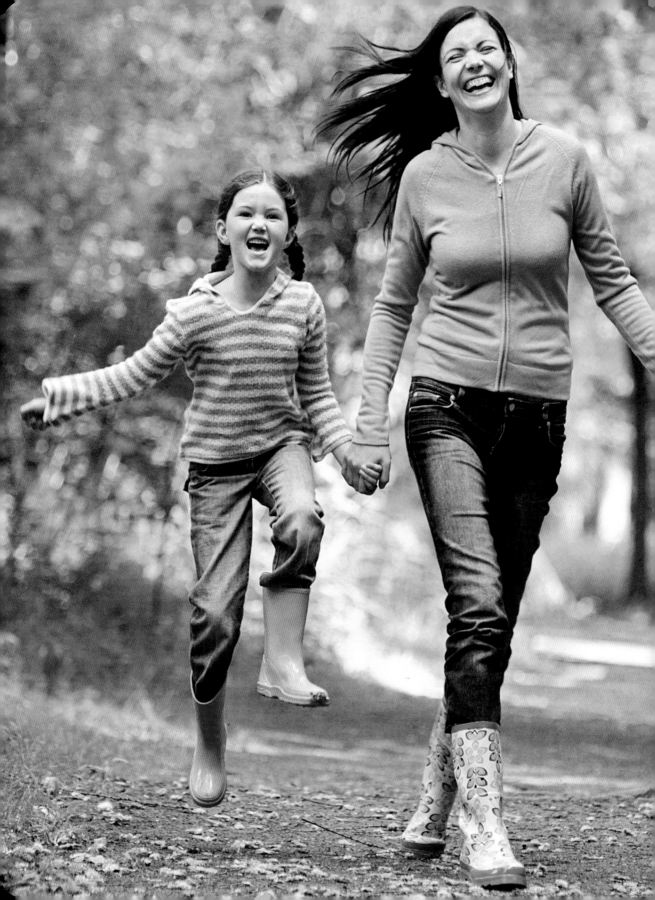

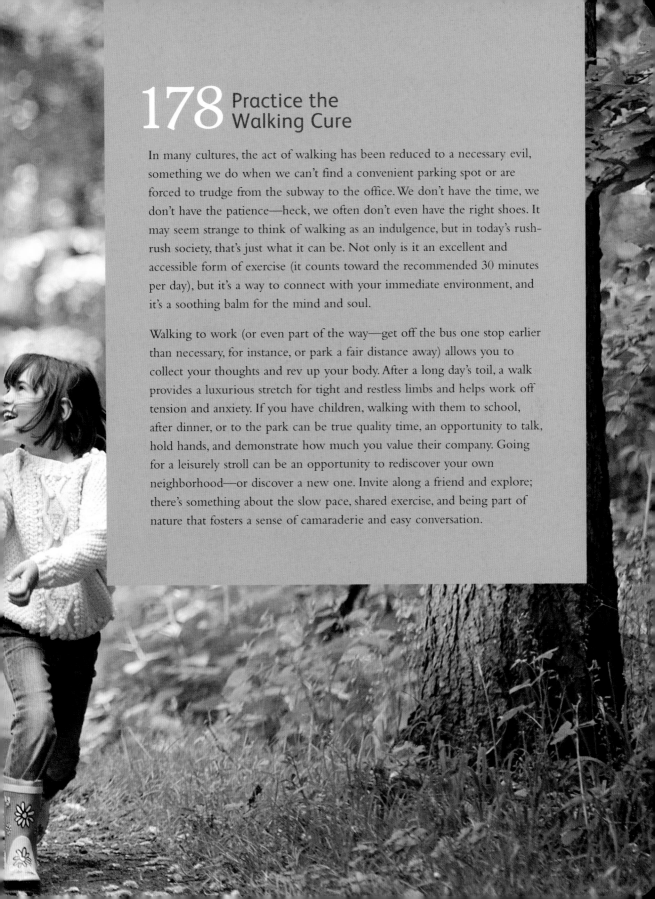

178 Practice the Walking Cure

In many cultures, the act of walking has been reduced to a necessary evil, something we do when we can't find a convenient parking spot or are forced to trudge from the subway to the office. We don't have the time, we don't have the patience—heck, we often don't even have the right shoes. It may seem strange to think of walking as an indulgence, but in today's rush-rush society, that's just what it can be. Not only is it an excellent and accessible form of exercise (it counts toward the recommended 30 minutes per day), but it's a way to connect with your immediate environment, and it's a soothing balm for the mind and soul.

Walking to work (or even part of the way—get off the bus one stop earlier than necessary, for instance, or park a fair distance away) allows you to collect your thoughts and rev up your body. After a long day's toil, a walk provides a luxurious stretch for tight and restless limbs and helps work off tension and anxiety. If you have children, walking with them to school, after dinner, or to the park can be true quality time, an opportunity to talk, hold hands, and demonstrate how much you value their company. Going for a leisurely stroll can be an opportunity to rediscover your own neighborhood—or discover a new one. Invite along a friend and explore; there's something about the slow pace, shared exercise, and being part of nature that fosters a sense of camaraderie and easy conversation.

179 Go Deep to Condition Your Hair

Treating hair with a warm oil base containing essential oils promotes shine and strength, helping combat the ill effects of blow-drying, chemical processes, and sun exposure.

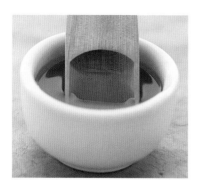

Deep-Conditioning Hair Treatment

1 teaspoon Brazil nut oil
1 teaspoon olive oil
1 teaspoon sesame oil
½ teaspoon honey
2 drops geranium essential oil
2 drops lavender essential oil

1 Mix the ingredients in the recipe at left in a small bowl or plastic bottle. Warm the oil mixture by setting the container in a large bowl or pan of hot water for a few minutes. (Heated oils can penetrate your hair better than unheated ones, making them more effective.)

2 After wetting your hair, rub the oil on your fingers and work it through your hair, starting at the top and moving down to the ends.

3 Soak a towel in warm water and wring it out, or put a damp towel in your dryer for a few minutes to warm it. Wrap the towel around your hair and leave it on for 5 to 15 minutes. (One of the advantages of a longer conditioning treatment is that it gives you time to take a relaxing bath, meditate, sit outdoors, or read a book.) Then wash your hair with your regular shampoo.

4 Comb your hair with a broad-toothed comb (brushes can break wet hair strands). Indulge in this treatment every few weeks—more often if your hair is very dry or damaged, less often if it's oily or fine.

180 Smooth Damaged Strands

Like nails, feathers, and even the baleen of whales, hair is a form of protein known as keratin. Human hair is strong—as strong as an iron wire, by some accounts—however, it can be damaged by chemical treatments, sunlight, chlorine, and rough handling. Use conditioning treatments to help the appearance of your hair when it's in bad shape. Damaged hair often has ruffled scales, and conditioners smooth those scales down, thus creating a smooth, shiny look.

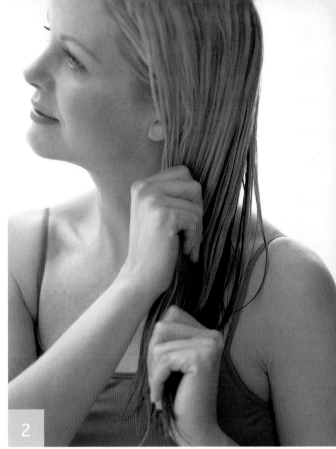

1

2

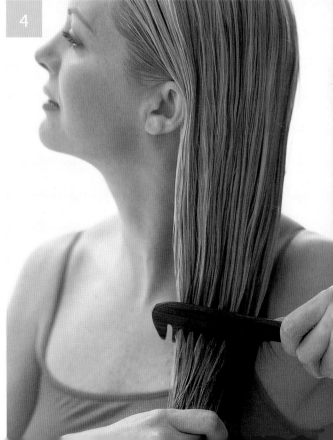

3

4

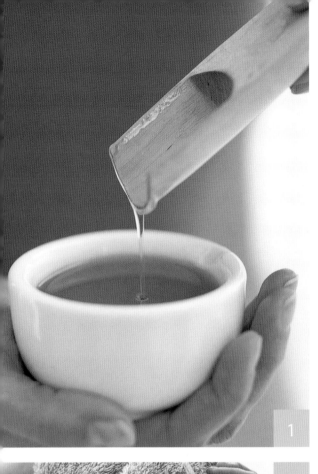

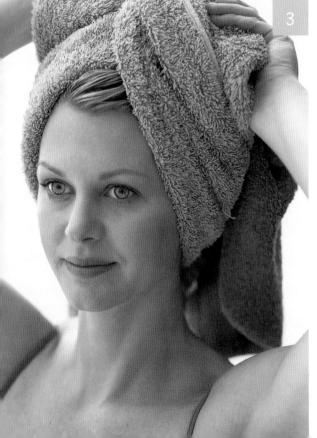

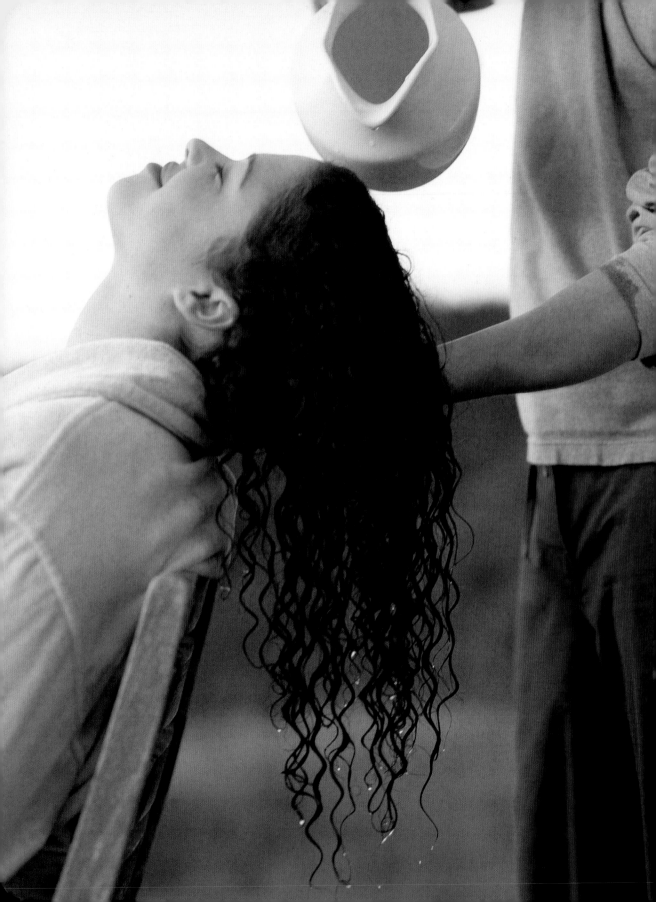

181 Share a Sensual Shampoo-for-Two

Taking turns shampooing each other's hair creates a cascade of sensual pleasures, while promoting an intimacy with your partner based on touch and care. The combination of fragrant shampoo, a gentle head massage, and the splash of warm water on your hair and scalp is a treat most of us get only at a salon. But letting a loved one wash your hair, and then switching places, is a wonderful way to indulge in caring for each other's well-being and connect emotionally. Start by creating a shampoo infused with your favorite essential oils (see the recipe at right). Then choose a relaxing spot for the shampooing—it might be in the shower, the bathtub, or even outside in the garden.

To begin, pour warm water over your partner's hair. Rub a little shampoo between your hands. Working slowly from the front hairline toward the crown and from the side hairlines to the back, massage the shampoo into the scalp and hair in small, circular movements. Try to move the scalp with your fingertips, but don't dig in too hard (that hurts) or rub the hair too roughly (that damages hair shafts). Make the shampooing a leisurely process; this is as much about connecting with your partner as it is about cleaning his or her hair. Rinse the hair thoroughly with warm water and pat it dry with a towel.

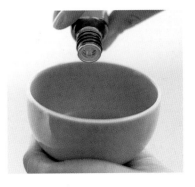

Sensual Shampoo Blend

6 to 8 ounces unscented shampoo
10 drops ylang-ylang essential oil
8 drops sandalwood essential oil
2 drops lavender essential oil

182 Work Up Just Enough Lather

A common misconception about shampoo is that its cleaning power is directly related to the amount of lather produced. Actually, some very fine, effective shampoos deliberately are formulated with lower amounts of detergent, the component that causes the lather. Too much detergent strips hair of its natural oils. Use a judicious amount of shampoo; unless your hair is very long or thick, a quarter-size dollop should do the job.

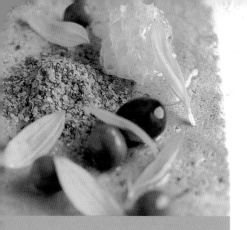

183

Cure Cuticles with Intensive Care

If your cuticles are truly in sorry shape, whip up an effective overnight treatment in your kitchen. Just before bedtime, blend one teaspoon of honey with one teaspoon of sunflower, wheat germ, or olive oil in a small bowl. Dip your fingers into the mix and massage it into the beds of your nails and cuticles. Cover your hands with cotton gloves or socks and leave on overnight.

184 Give Yourself a Healthy-Hand Manicure

Parched skin? Uneven or brittle nails? Unruly cuticles? It's time to give your hardworking hands a little TLC with a manicure designed to make them look and feel good.

1 Begin your manicure by filling a medium-size bowl with warm water. Add two drops of lavender essential oil; the lavender acts as a soothing, antibacterial agent, helping to clean and disinfect nail beds (it smells wonderful, too). Immerse the tips of your fingers in the water, ensuring that your nails and cuticles are completely covered. Soak your fingers for at least five minutes to soften the cuticles and prime your nails for the remaining steps.

2 Using an emery board, file each nail to form a pleasing shape and eliminate any ragged edges. Start from one side and, in one smooth movement, draw the file toward the center of the nail several times; then repeat on the other side. Be careful not to saw back and forth, which can cause nails to splinter. After you've finished filing your nails, gently push back the cuticles using an orange stick wrapped in a small piece of cotton. (Never cut your cuticles, as cutting can increase the risk of an infection.) Following the natural contours of your nails, try to expose as much of the nail surface as possible to give each one a long, elegant silhouette.

3 Your hands have fewer oil glands than the rest of your body and are prone to dryness and premature aging. Apply a restorative hand cream, such as one containing vitamin E, to keep them hydrated. Also use a broad-spectrum sunscreen with an SPF of 30 or higher on your hands every day to help keep wrinkles and age spots at bay.

4 Use a buffing file or block to give your nails a natural shine. Hold the buffing tool between your thumb and fingers while you curl the fingers of your other hand in toward your palm. Extend one finger at a time, and apply the buffer in a back-and-forth motion across each nail. Use quick, smooth strokes to give nails a healthy, polished look.

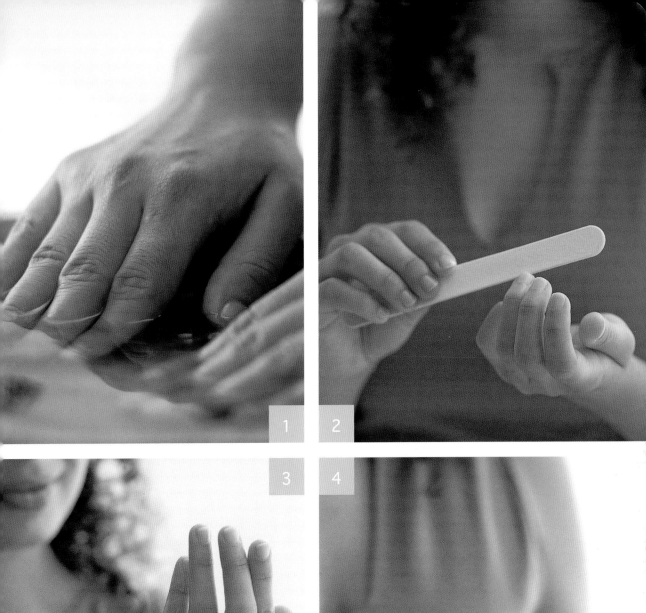
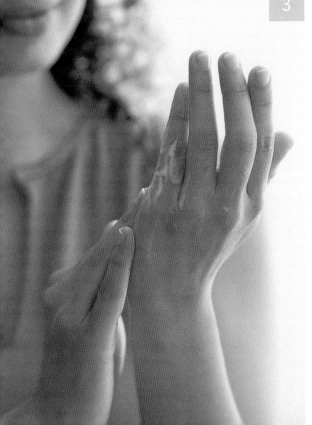
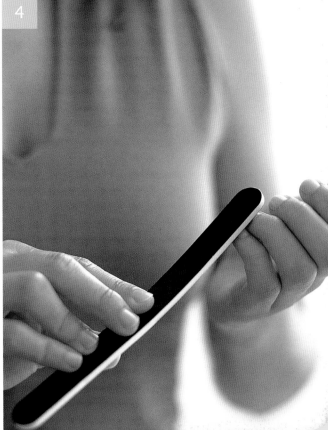

1

2

3

4

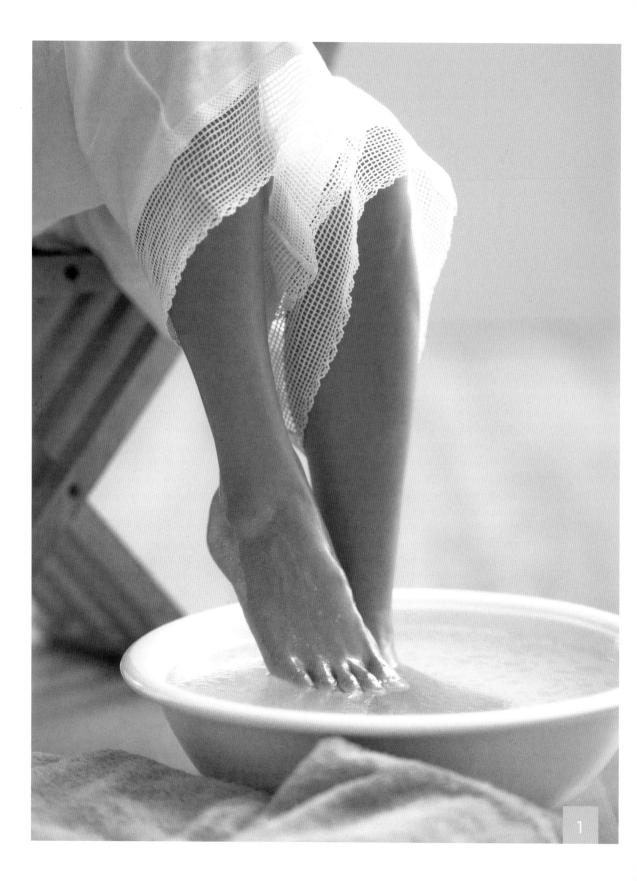

185 Help Yourself to Hydrated Feet

Indulge your feet in a moisturizing soak, some judicious heel-filing, and an overnight hydrating. This treatment can work wonders on them, especially if your skin tends to be dry or rough.

1 Fill a bowl large enough to immerse your feet completely with warm water, then add five drops of neroli essential oil and three tablespoons of olive oil and mix well. Neroli's floral fragrance is relaxing and uplifting; olive oil is known for its softening, emollient properties. Soak your feet for 15 minutes, then rest them on a towel.

2 While your feet are still damp, use a firm back-and-forth motion with a foot file or pumice stone to remove the dead skin that tends to accumulate on the heels, balls of the feet, and bottoms of big toes. Check every few strokes to feel your skin; when it no longer feels rough in a certain area, move on to the next problem spot. (And, of course, stop at any sign of pain.) If your feet are severely dry and cracked, it might take several treatments to smooth them.

3 Hydrate your newly exposed fresh skin. For dramatic results, slather your feet with an intensive moisturizer, such as hemp oil, then slip on a pair of deep-moisturizing foot booties or cotton socks and leave them on overnight.

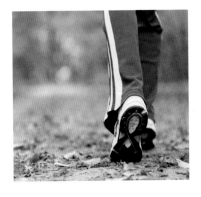

Get Shoes Fit for Your Feet

When buying shoes, reward your feet by making comfort and support priorities. Our feet are intricate structures consisting of 26 bones, 30 muscles, and 114 ligaments. Human feet take a pounding of 10,000 steps daily, on average, with each of those steps subjecting these relatively small structures to about three times our weight.

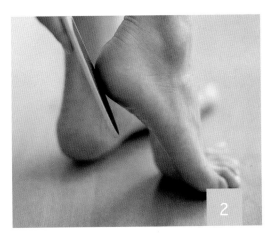

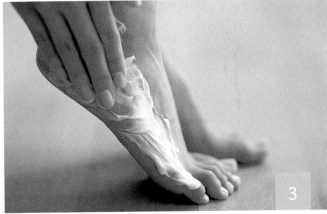

186 Cocoon Yourself in a Blanket Wrap

Try topping off a luxurious bath soak with a period of rest under warm blankets. Bath or no bath, a restful wrap is a nice escape when you need a little quiet cocooning time. During this rest period, your parasympathetic nervous system works its restorative magic, slowing down your heart rate, regulating the digestion of food, and generally helping your body run more smoothly and efficiently.

To prepare for your restful wrap, spread two or three heavy blankets on your bed; use a soft blanket on top, as it will be the layer in contact with your body. Place one or two pillows on the bed, so you can rest your head at a comfortable height and angle. Remove all of your clothing, lie on the blankets, and wrap them snugly around your body. Rest with your eyes closed for 20 to 30 minutes. Use the time to meditate, remember the positive events of the day, fantasize about your next vacation—anything but worry.

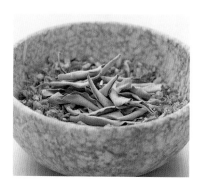

Restful Wrap Spray-Mist Blend

1 cup distilled water
2 drops jasmine essential oil
1 drop clary sage essential oil

187 Add Luxury to a Blanket Wrap

For an indulgent variation on a blanket wrap, use a spray-mister to scent the blankets used in your wrap with your favorite essential oils. In our restful blend (see recipe at left) we included clary sage (the dried leaves pictured), which aromatherapists use as an antidote to depression and anxiety—it also has a reputation as something of an aphrodisiac. Jasmine (the dried flowers pictured) is thought to relieve anxiety, stress, and depression, as well as bolster the libido.

If you prefer, just spray a bath towel with the essential-oil blend and place that on top of the blankets instead (it's easier to wash the scent out of a towel than a pile of blankets). In cool weather, you also can heat up your wrap by spraying a little water on your bath towel or the top blanket and tumbling it in the dryer for about ten minutes right before you place it on the bed. To make the soothing heat last even longer, place a hot-water bottle or heating pad in the wrap.

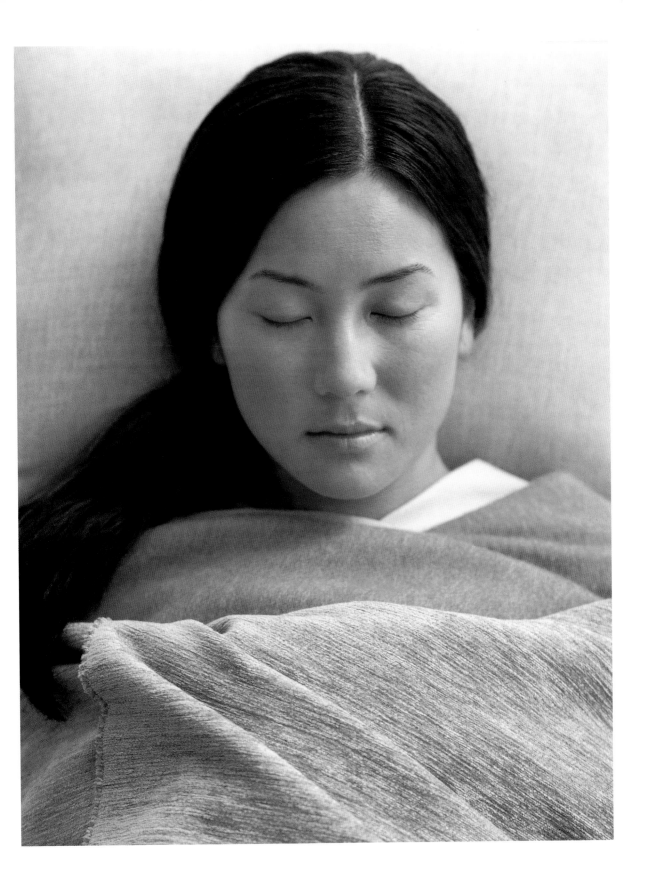

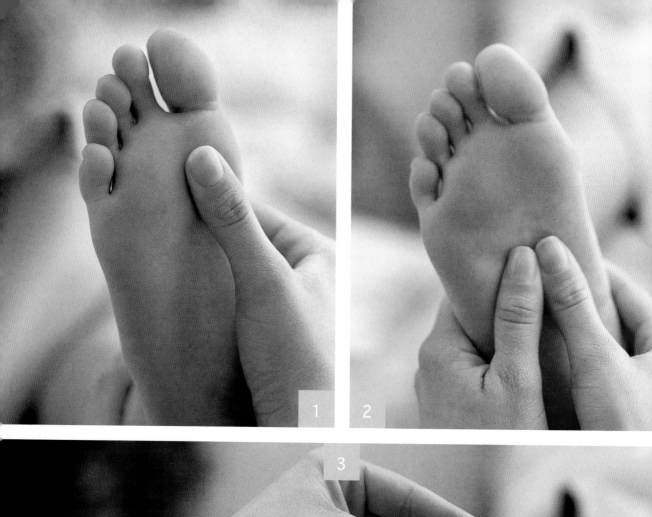

1　2

3

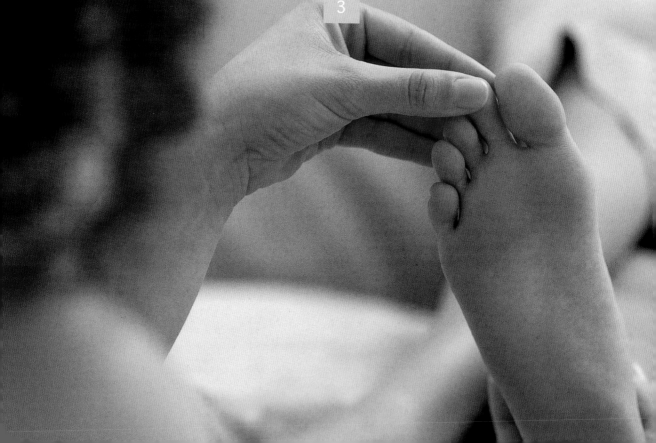

188 Get in the Zone with Foot Reflexology

Reflexologists believe zones in the feet exert beneficial influences on other body parts when pressed. A foot massage also ranks among life's simple pleasures. Recruit a friend to treat you to these soothing steps:

1 Get into a comfortable position for massaging your friend's foot. To activate the reflexology zones, begin by using your thumb to make deep, overlapping circles over the entire surface of her heel and arch. Then place your thumb just above her arch at the base of the ball of the foot and press into one of the grooves between the bones that lead up to the toes. Circle with your thumb up each groove, moving from the top of the arch toward each toe.

2 Grip her foot with both hands, with thumbs holding the bottom of the foot at mid-heel level. With your thumbs braced side by side for firm pressure, glide up her sole to the grooves in the ball of the foot and then up to the space between the big and second toes. Ease your grip and slide lightly back to her heel. Repeat two more times.

3 Give each toe an individual massage by pressing your thumb and index finger together and circling from base to tip. Then wiggle each toe backward, forward, and around in circles, starting with small circles and spiraling into bigger ones, being careful not to bend the toes too far. For a soothing finish, do a foot sweep: Contour and press your hands together on the top and bottom of your friend's foot. Gently pull your hands toward you and off her toes three times. Then repeat all these massage steps on the other foot.

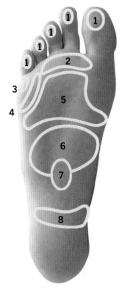

Right Foot Reflexology Map

Here are some of the key reflexology points on the sole of your right foot:

1 Sinus, head, and brain
2 Eyes and ears
3 Arms
4 Shoulders
5 Lungs and breasts
6 Liver
7 Kidneys
8 Sciatic nerve

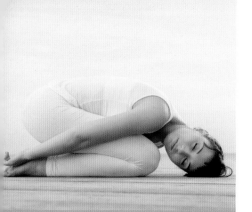

189

Unleash Trapped Emotions

In some yoga traditions, the hips are considered the seat of emotional vulnerability. This means that as you release physical tension in this area, you also might experience the release of pent-up emotions, such as fear, anger, or sorrow. That can be a bit unsettling, but if you let these feelings rise, wash over you, and pass, you'll appreciate the relief that comes with detaching yourself from emotions (rather than clinging to them), as well as the clarity that comes from releasing them.

190 Rock the Tension Out of Your Body

Releasing tension in the hip joints with Rock the Baby pose soothes and stretches your back. Dissipating the physical tension can offer surprising emotional rewards as well.

Sit with your legs extended in front of you. Bend your right knee and lift your right leg toward your chest. Keeping your back as straight as possible, hug your leg inward and gently rock it from side to side, the same way you'd rock a baby. Ideally, your elbows will wrap around your knee and foot, but use any grasp that feels comfortable. As you rock, take four to eight deep breaths. Repeat the pose with your other leg.

While you're doing this or other yoga poses that stretch the hips, focus on your second chakra—one of seven spots in the body where yogis believe channels of energy intersect. The second chakra, located just below the navel, governs creativity, sexuality, fertility, and sensuality, as well as emotions such as anger, fear, and the instinct to nurture. Yogis believe that the second chakra, when well balanced (that is, not blocked or overactive), can help women feel more powerful, creative, and sensual.

191 Loosen Hips to Help Your Back

It's well known that poor posture, incorrect lifting techniques, and sedentary lifestyles can contribute to lower-back pain. What few of us realize, however, is that sometimes those back problems actually are rooted in the hips. That's because chronic sitting (in your car or at your desk, for instance) can result in shortened hip flexors—the muscles at the front of your hips. Even certain exercises, such as stair climbing, leg lifts, and bicycling, can tighten the hip flexors. To help avoid back problems, try to include stretching your hip flexors in your fitness routine and work on maintaining a full range of motion in the hips.

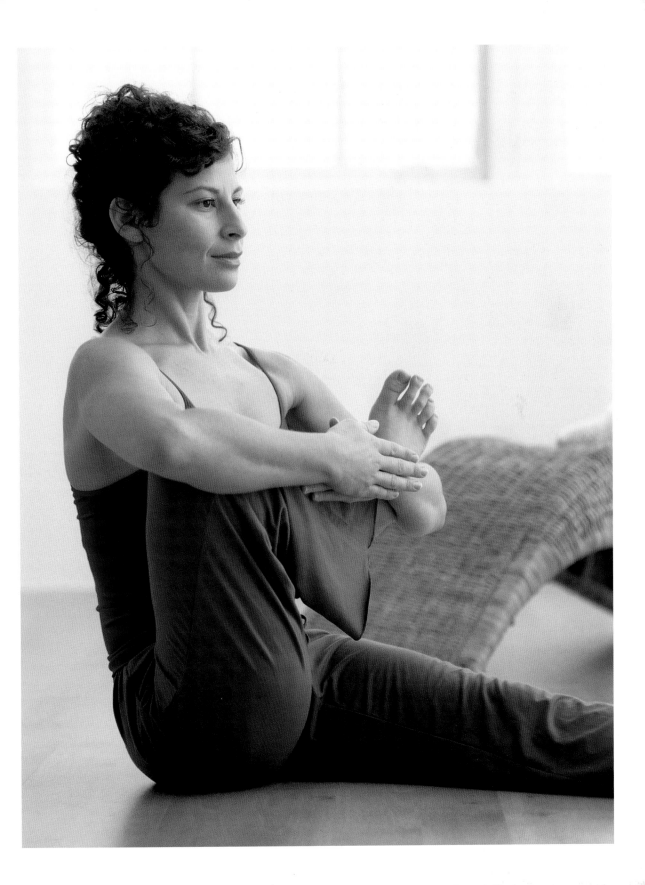

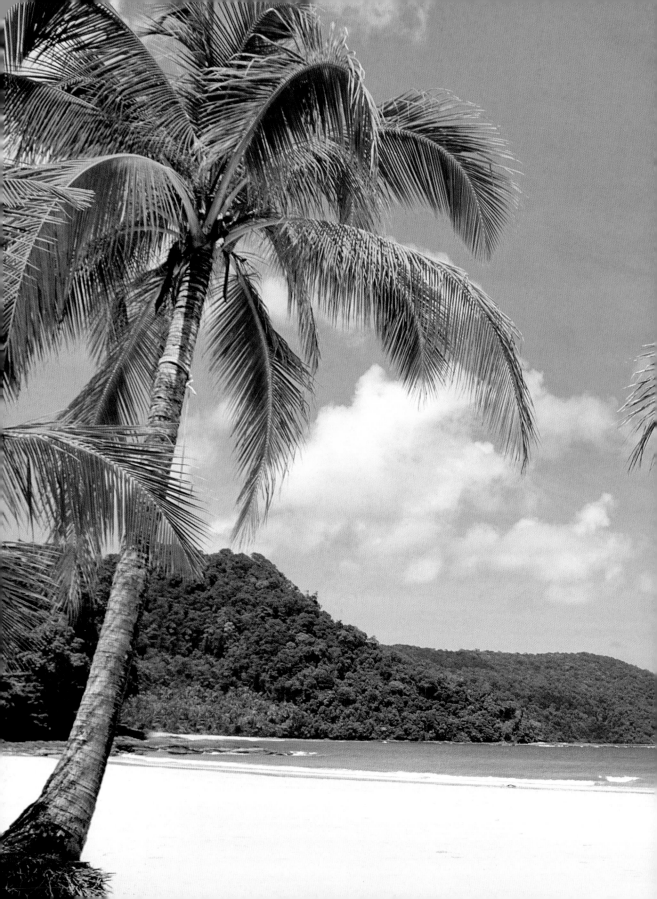

192 Visualize a Peaceful Haven

Find a place where you can count on being undisturbed for ten minutes or so. Sit in a comfortable chair, and rest your forearms and hands lightly in your lap or on the arms of the chair. Close your eyes. Begin breathing slowly and deeply. Let go of any thoughts racing through your mind—the need to call the vet or a work deadline. Just concentrate on the regular rise and fall of your breath. Start by focusing on the soles of your feet and work your way slowly up to the small muscles in your scalp, consciously relaxing your entire body and applying only enough muscle control to keep you sitting upright in your chair.

Now you're ready for your great escape. Visualize your favorite setting, a beautiful place where you feel happy and totally at ease. For many people, that special venue involves the curve of a white-sand beach lapped by a serene, azure sea. Picture yourself walking along the beach. Feel the soft, powdery sand crunching under your feet and the gentle breeze ruffling your hair. Listen to the steady rhythm of the waves, and enjoy the heady fragrance of the tropical flowers that grow just beyond the sandy shores. Set your towel and stretch out in the sunshine. When you're ready, stand, pick up your towel, and head for home, knowing that you can return to your solitary paradise any time you wish.

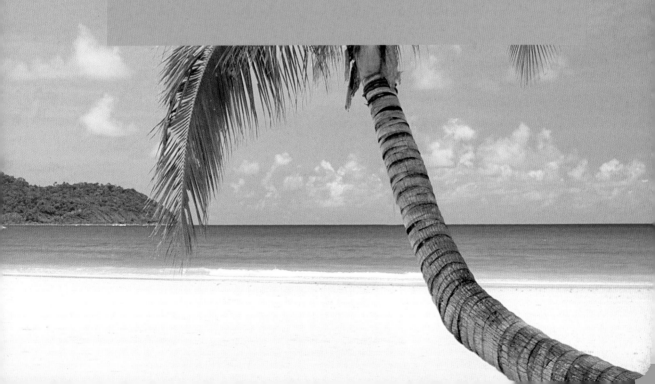

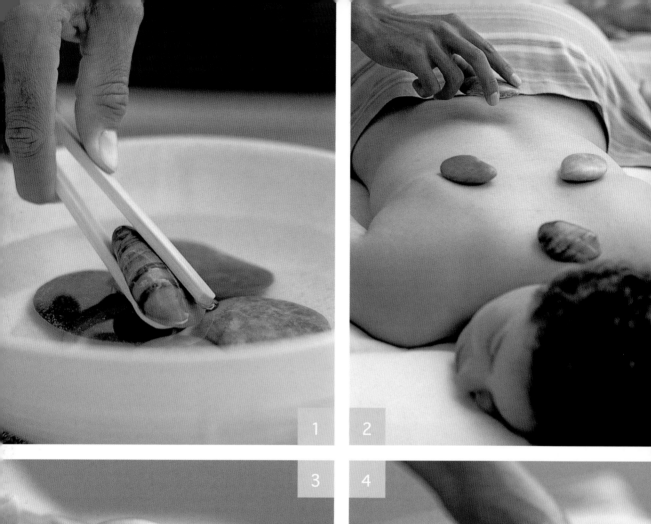

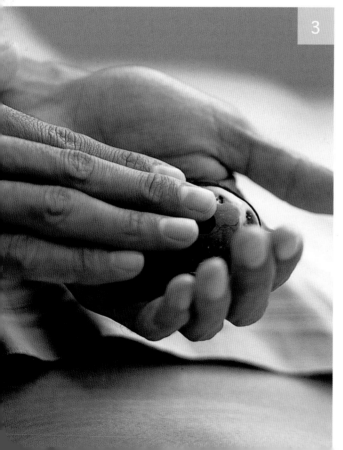

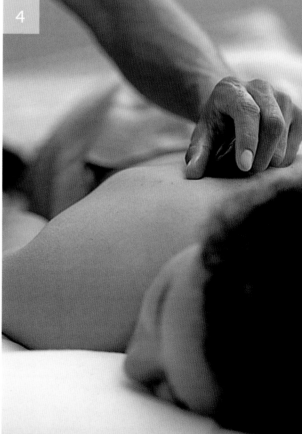

1

2

3

4

193 Feel the Soothing Heat of a Hot-Stone Massage

Placed on key energy points and used as massage tools, hot stones can help you and your loved one relax and give you a new way to touch each other. Provide your partner with these massage instructions, as you prepare for your treatment by lying facedown on a bed or a comfortable mat on the floor, with your arms at your sides and your palms facing up:

1 Put seven flat, smooth, clean stones in a large bowl or pan and cover them with boiling water. Heat them for five to ten minutes. Using tongs, remove the stones from the hot water one at a time and dry each as you're about to place it on your partner. Test the temperature of the stones with your hand to be sure that they're not too hot. Start by placing a stone in each of your partner's palms.

2 Place one stone on the muscles next to each shoulder blade, and another stone at the base of her neck. Finish with a stone gently placed at the base of her spine. Allow your partner to rest for ten minutes, so she can feel the warmth and heft of the stones stimulate energy points and help coax away her tension.

3 Once the stones have cooled, take them away in the order in which you placed them. Then remove the remaining stone from the hot water and dry it off. Hold it in the palm of your hand and pour a little massage oil on it, rubbing the stone between your hands to cover it with the oil. For added pleasure, add three drops of rose, jasmine, or ylang-ylang essential oil to the massage oil.

4 Use one of the smooth edges of the warm, oiled stone to gently massage your partner's back. Placing the stone on one side of the base of her spine (never press directly on the spine), glide it upward with light pressure in one smooth movement. Stroke up to, and then along, the inside of the right shoulder blade. Repeat this gliding stroke twice more, gradually increasing the amount of pressure but not rubbing too hard. Now repeat on the other side of her back.

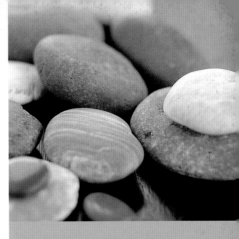

194 Choose the Right Rocks

You can find rocks suitable for massage at craft stores, or collect them from a beach or riverbed. Select ones that have a bit of weight to them but are not so heavy that they would cause discomfort when placed on your partner's body.

195 Spice Up the Atmosphere with Potpourri

A perennial aromatherapy favorite, lovely bags or bowls of delicious scents can spice up a room, sweeten a friendship, or even evoke memories and moods. Potpourri is a combination of aromatic and decorative ingredients, such as dried flower petals, leaves, fruits, spices, and wood shavings, sprinkled with essential oils. Better-quality potpourri also contains fixatives, such as orrisroot, that absorb and slowly release the essential oils, helping the fragrance last longer. You can purchase ready-made potpourri at gift and craft stores, but you might find it more rewarding to create your own special blend.

First, find a potpourri recipe that sounds appealing; look in books, browse online, or try the recipe at left. Craft shops, herb catalogs, and natural-food stores will have the ingredients you need (as might your own backyard), but you'll also need a few tools, such as clean glass jars, a kitchen scale (for measuring ingredients), and glass eyedroppers (one for each oil you use). Be forewarned: Making potpourri doesn't take much time, but the mix has to settle for about three weeks before it's ready to use, so plan ahead if you're making gifts.

Once your mixture is ready, you can put it in pretty bowls and place them strategically throughout your home (avoid using very strongly scented potpourri near where you're eating, because it can interfere with the taste of your food). You also can make sachets by placing potpourri in small bags of porous cloth, such as linen, cotton, or silk, tied with ribbons; these impart a delicate scent to your clothes when placed in closets or dresser drawers.

To really unleash the aroma of your mixture, sprinkle the potpourri in a pot of water and simmer it on the stove. Besides these purely atmospheric uses, potpourri can serve practical purposes: Ingredients such as rosemary, citronella, sage, cedar, and lavender help repel moths, for example, while a mixture of chamomile, bergamot, lavender, and clary sage placed at your bedside helps promote a good night's sleep.

Induce Peace Through Scent

Make a comforting potpourri from a mixture of dried orange rinds and lavender, rose, and jasmine petals—perfect on your nightstand or desk. A few drops of the corresponding essential oils will help make the fragrance more pronounced and longer-lasting.

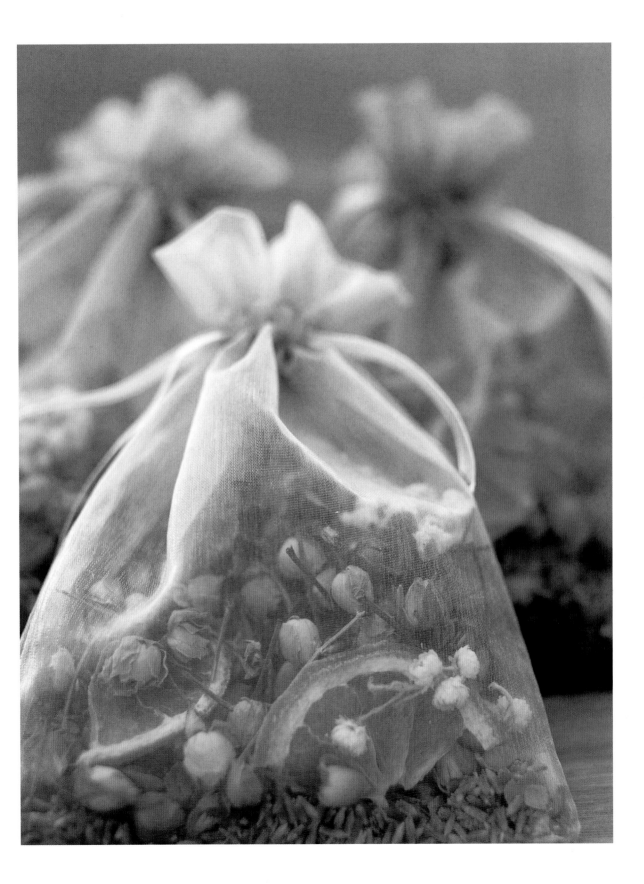

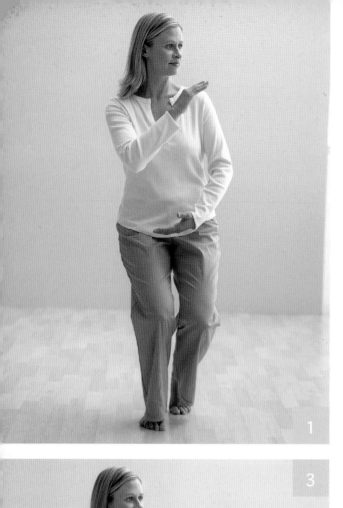

1

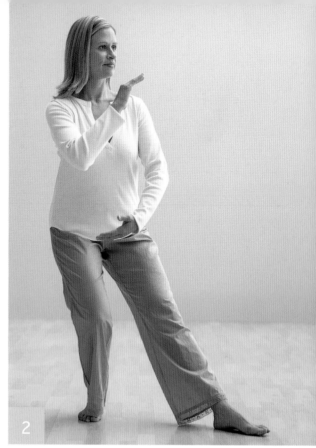

2

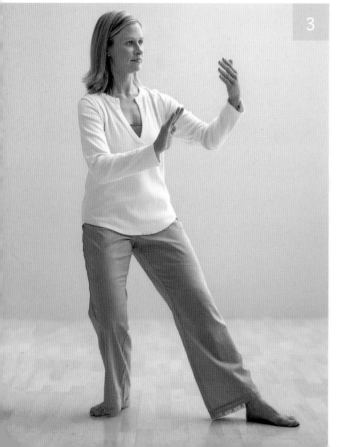

3

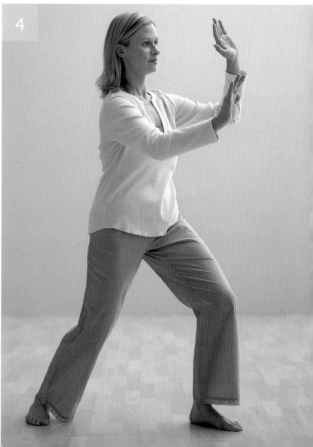

4

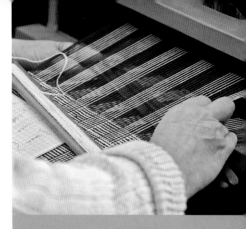

196 Honor Yourself with Tai Chi

This soothing tai chi sequence, Fair Lady Works at Shuttles, honors women's handiwork and service. The movements are traditionally repeated four times in four different directions.

1 Stand with your left foot behind your right foot, knees slightly bent and positioned directly over your toes. Lift your right arm across your body to about shoulder height, with the elbow bent and the palm facing down. Then bring your left arm down below your belly button, keeping the elbow bent and the palm up. Keep your elbows, wrists, and knees soft; that is, don't form any hard angles at the joints.

2 Step out with your left foot, sinking your weight onto the right foot. Keep your arms round, with the right hand still above the left.

3 Roll your hips back as you move your left arm up (with the palm now facing in). Draw your right arm back, palm now facing out.

4 Push both hands out in front of you until the left arm is above your right arm and the fingers are tipped slightly back. Shift your weight to follow the hands' movements and bend your left knee. Repeat Steps 1 through 4 three more times.

197 Stay Soft and Feel the Energy

The idea of maintaining softness in your body is a very important principle when practicing tai chi. Keep your arms and legs loose and curved, taking care not to fully extend them. Pay special attention to your hands, which should always be soft. When you move through a tai chi sequence, position your hands with intention and imagine sending your inner energy out to the very tips of your fingers.

198 Turn Four Times

The name of this tai chi sequence, Fair Lady Works at Shuttles, comes from the Chinese legend of a serving maid weaving at four looms belonging to the Taoist immortals. Picture yourself moving tirelessly from shuttle to shuttle, as you repeat the meditative movements four times in four different directions. The four directions reflect the ancient Chinese belief that the world is square and the heavens are supported by a tortoise's four legs, which represent the four points of the compass, too.

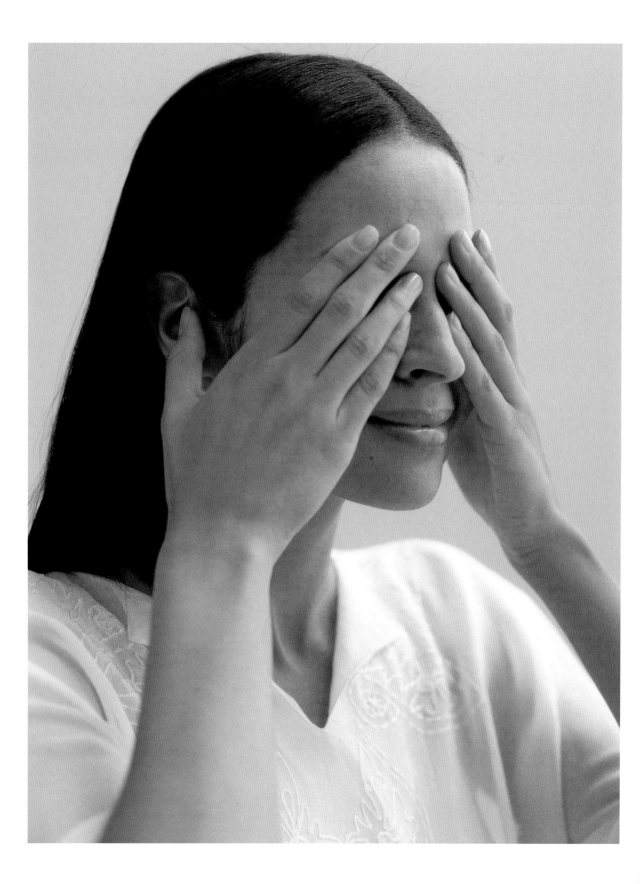

199 Hum Like a Bee to Buzz Away Tension

The pleasing, audible vibration in this yoga breathing practice helps to clarify the mind and calm the spirit. Easy to do, it can be enjoyed by children and adults. Called the *bhramari pranayama* in Sanskrit, the Humming Bee Breath can help you with your meditation, as well as help relieve tension, dispel anger, lower blood pressure, and soothe insomnia. It is a wonderful exercise for those times when you need to calm yourself—or a small child (or both).

- Sit in a comfortable meditation pose with your back straight. Place your hands over your eyes.

- Use your thumbs to press down gently on the *tragi,* the little flaps at the front of your ears, so that they seal off the openings to the ear canals. (The idea is to cut off external sensory inputs.)

- Inhale deeply. Then exhale slowly through your nostrils while at the same time humming high in the back of your mouth, so you feel a vibration on your soft palate (the fleshy back part of the roof of your mouth). Lengthen each exhalation, drawing it out as long as you can.

- Practice for three to seven breaths; then release, close your eyes, rest your hands on your knees, and enjoy the quiet state of mind that you have created.

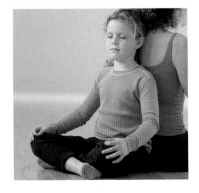

Start Yoga Young

By practicing yoga, adults and children alike can become more aware of their bodies and emotions, relax more easily, and cultivate the ability to concentrate. Yoga also helps all of us develop better coordination, posture, and balance. To help keep a younger practitioner focused as you practice, try talking about what's happening with your bodies or counting together.

200 Enjoy the Benefits of Abdominal Breathing

Unless instructed otherwise, abdominal breathing is a good, all-round technique to use in yoga class. In fact, whether you're practicing yoga or jogging, using your diaphragm to breathe more deeply can increase the efficiency of each breath. To get the hang of abdominal breathing, sit in a comfortable position and place one hand on your abdomen just below your rib cage. Expand your abdomen when you inhale, then contract it when you exhale. Continue for about five minutes.

201 Comfort a Friend with Energy Holds

Inspired by Ayurvedic chakra work and other ancient forms of healing, these moves allow a friend or partner to connect with you through the power of touch. Have that person treat you to these comforting energy holds by following these four simple steps:

1 Have your friend lie faceup. Briskly rub your hands together for about 20 seconds to help warm them. Place your hands under your friend's head, with your thumbs above her ears and the rest of your fingers beneath. Don't press down; just hold her head lightly for a minute or so to help her relax as she lies comfortably on her back.

2 Rest your right hand below her navel and your left hand on her forehead. Keeping your left hand still, rock your right hand from side to side, using enough pressure to gently rock her hips from side to side. Rock her for 20 seconds, then rest for 20 seconds, keeping your hands in place. Alternate rocking and resting for a few minutes.

3 Have your friend roll over onto her stomach. Place one of your hands on the top of her tailbone and the other hand at the base of her neck. Gently rock her hips from side to side with your lower hand for 20 seconds; then be still for 20 seconds, keeping both hands in place. Repeat this cycle for a few minutes until her breathing becomes deep, calm, and regular.

4 Place one of your hands over the other a few inches above her lower back for a moment. You're tapping into an energy field that many traditional healers believe radiates from the body. Then set your hands lightly on her back and rock gently, alternating between rocking and stillness. Be sensitive to any sense of warmth or tingling—signs of pent-up energy being released. After five full breaths, slowly lift your hands, and hold them a few inches above her body for another moment.

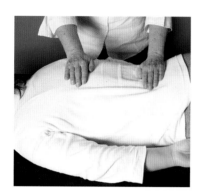

Heal with Charged Hands

Many energy healers believe that we have a slightly positive charge in our right hand and a slightly negative charge in our left hand. When we touch someone with both hands, the difference in charges supposedly causes a mild but potent electrical current to flow between the hands. This current is thought to help break up any energy blockages in the person we're touching, allowing his or her own energy to flow freely and helping to restore balance, health, and well-being.

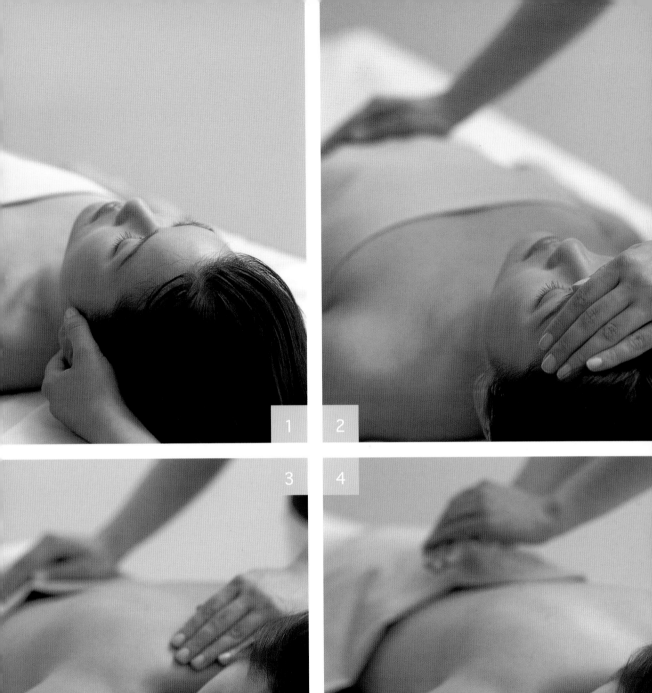

1

2

3

4

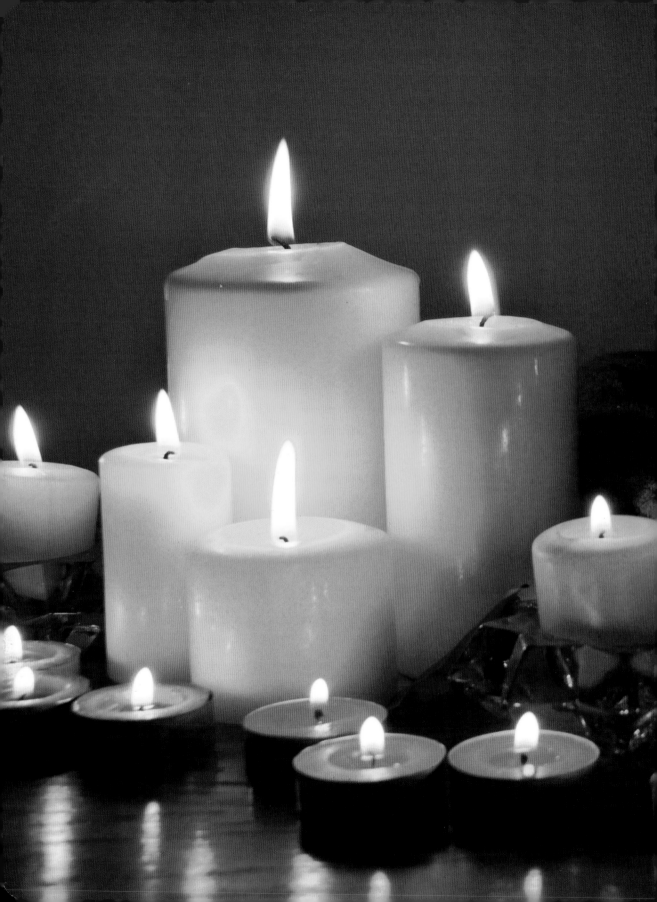

202 Set the Mood with Flickering Candles

The soft, dancing light provided by candles can create an enchanting and alluring environment. Placing a few or even a whole collection of candles throughout a room can transform it into a lovely, magical space in just a matter of minutes: Your kitchen suddenly feels like an atmospheric café, your bathroom a luxurious spa, and, perhaps most dramatic, your bedroom a mysterious and seductive hideaway.

If you'd like to enjoy the benefits of aromatherapy, place a few drops of essential oil on an unscented candle, near its wick. As the wax melts, the aroma will be released. Remember that essential oils are flammable; don't use too much or put them directly on a burning wick. In the bedroom, you might try using the oil from ylang-ylang flowers; it's reputed both to be an aphrodisiac and to alleviate performance anxieties, as does vetiver, which is known as "the oil of tranquility." Candles scented with jasmine, patchouli, neroli, sandalwood, frankincense, geranium, or rose are also thought to put one in the mood for love.

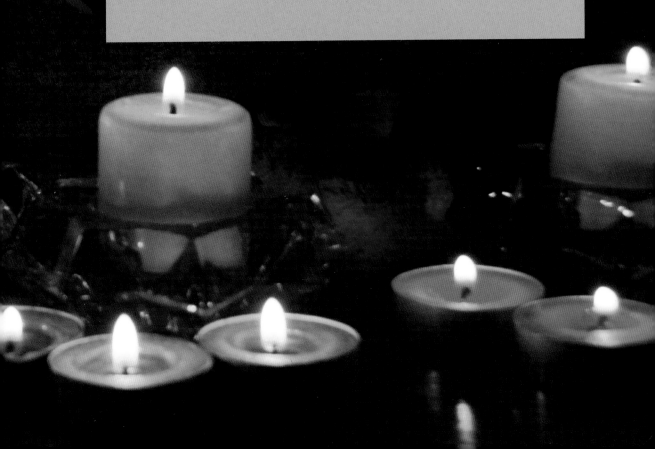

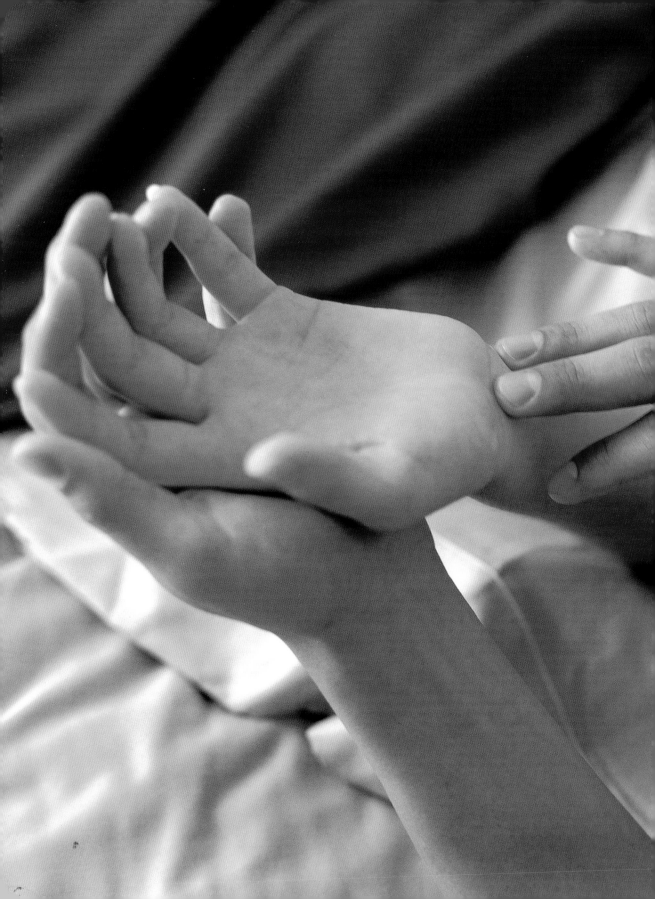

203 Caress Each Other with Sensual Massage

Get ready to turn up the heat with a loving massage. The light strokes and attention to sensitive zones let your partner explore you in an especially intimate way. Begin this massage with you and your partner resting comfortably in bed. Lay your back against your partner's chest, and ask him to follow these sensual massage steps:

1 Start by stroking along her forehead, between her eyebrows, circling down along the cheekbones, and moving across to the bridge of the nose. Slip your fingers down to your partner's lips; outline and explore them with the gentlest touch. Then circle around her ears, lightly tracing the outer rims and inner surfaces.

2 Continue your gentle caresses by stroking the soft, sensitive skin of your partner's inner arms, elbows, and forearms. Take your partner's hand in yours and softly stroke the wrist and hand all the way to the end of each fingertip. Repeat on the other hand.

3 Move to the navel, and slowly trace your fingertips across the belly and along the hips. Then trace inward along the waist to the navel. Circle the navel a few times, and glide up the belly to the breastbone. Continue to explore, lingering to circle sensitive spots.

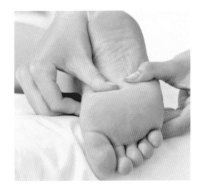

Rub Your Partner the Right Way

As you massage your loved one, experiment to find just the right amount of pleasing pressure. You want to use light, easy sweeps in this sensual exercise, but if you stroke too softly, you risk tickling, not titillating, your partner.

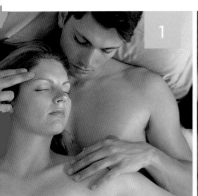
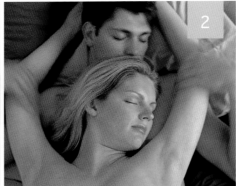
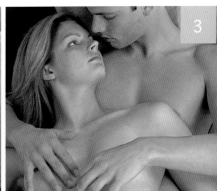

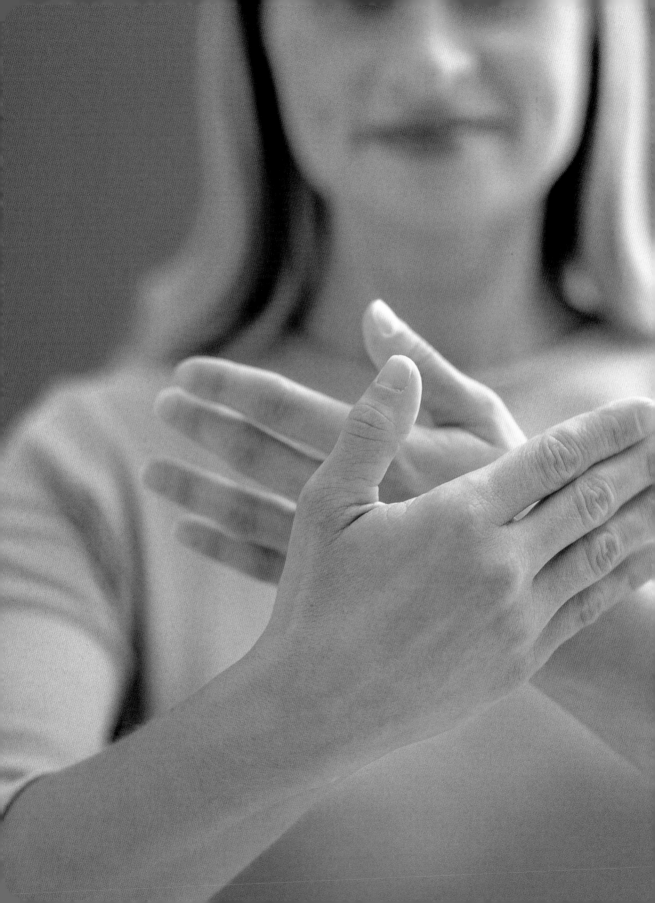

204 Wind Down with Tai Chi's Closing Sequence

Feeling wound up? We all have had that feeling of having too much pent-up energy rocketing around in our bodies—that anxious sense of having been overstimulated, overcaffeinated, or just generally overwrought by the course of the day's events.

While performing tai chi should help you relax, not make you feel anxious, tai chi practitioners still believe that it is important to settle down the body's chi (or energy) after completing a form (a series of tai chi movements). That's because this ancient internal and martial art focuses on gathering and stimulating the flow of chi. If that energy isn't calmed, however, it can leave the tai chi practitioner feeling scattered or not centered.

The flowing arm movements in the Closing Sequence (see next page) are believed to help push the chi down and settle it. If you're having trouble picturing this, think of smoothing out wrinkled sheets or a slightly mussed tablecloth. Some tai chi practitioners compare these movements to those of the setting sun. In whatever way you envision them, remember this: The overriding goal is to preserve the energy in the body and, at the same time, to relax the energy in a calm, meditative fashion.

205 Enjoy the Benefits of Tai Chi

Tai chi's fluid, weight-shifting movements help strengthen leg muscles, maintain bone density, enhance joint flexibility, and promote a good sense of balance and body awareness. You'll probably feel more relaxed and graceful after your first couple of weeks of tai chi sessions, but keep it up for a few months and you'll likely experience even greater results.

206 Find Calmness with Tai Chi

Feel your mind quiet and your body relax as you do the soothing, meditative moves of the tai chi Closing Sequence. Try it after an exercise session or a long day of work.

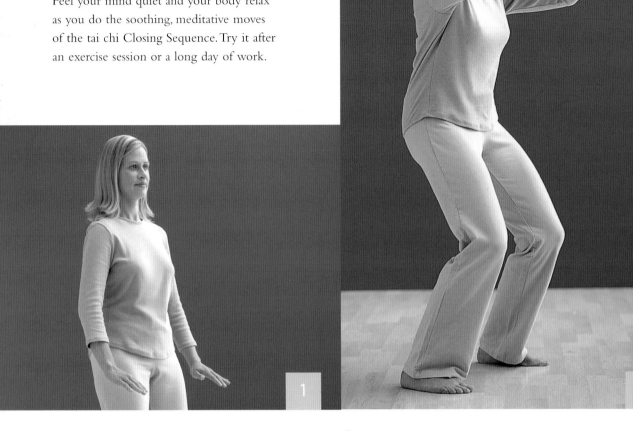

1

1 Stand with your feet shoulder-width apart and toes pointing straight ahead. Start with your arms relaxed by your sides. Go into a shallow squat, keeping your tailbone tucked in, eyes straight ahead, and knees relaxed. As you sink, start to raise your hands.

2 Breathing easily and naturally, keep raising your hands until they are chin height, with your palms facing out. Slowly move your arms down and out in a large circle, keeping your eyes focused straight ahead.

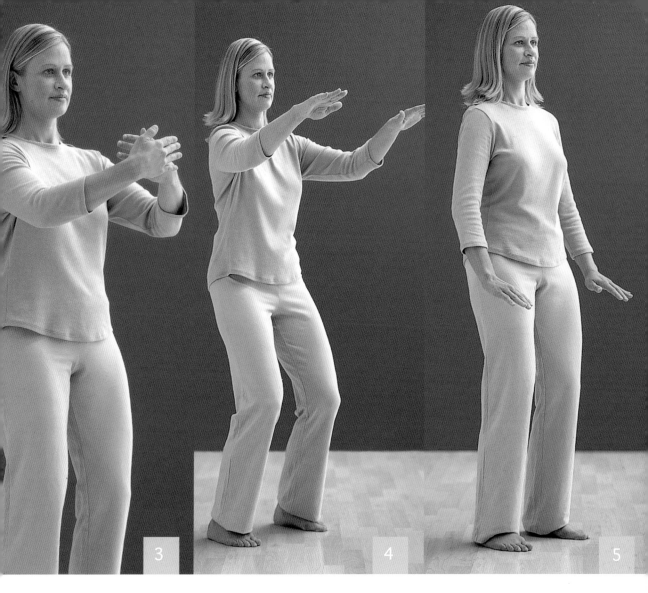

3 3 Now bring your hands
down and together, so they
cross in front of your body at
about shoulder height but do
not touch each other. Turn
your palms toward you.

4 4 Turn your palms to face the
ground and begin to stretch
your hands out in front of you,
as if you're pushing them along
the surface of a table. Drop
and relax your shoulders.

5 5 Keeping your feet hip-
width apart, rise out of the
squat and let your arms sink
down and rest by your sides.
End by taking a step in with
one foot. Repeat Steps 1
through 5 four times.

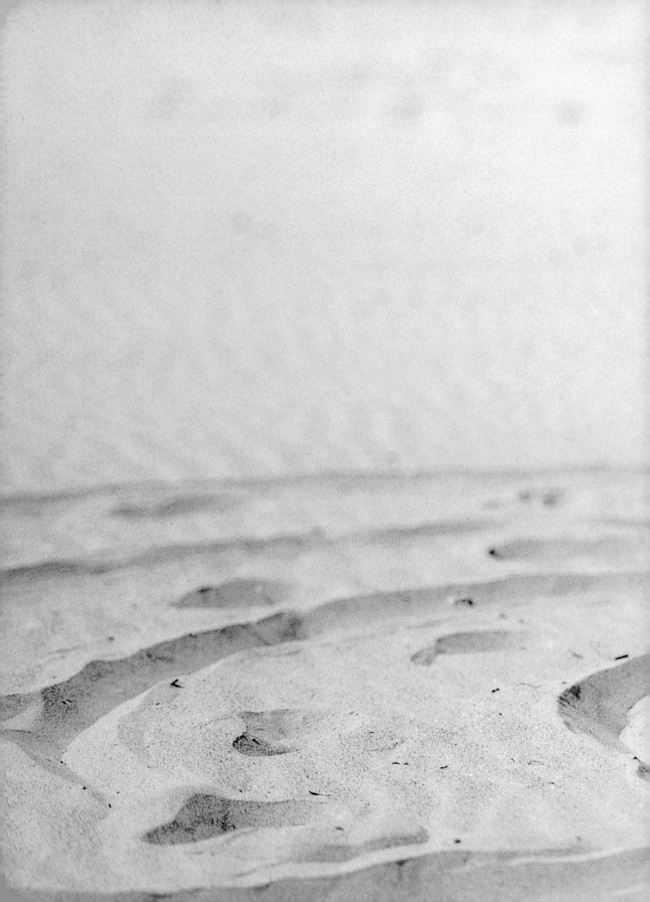

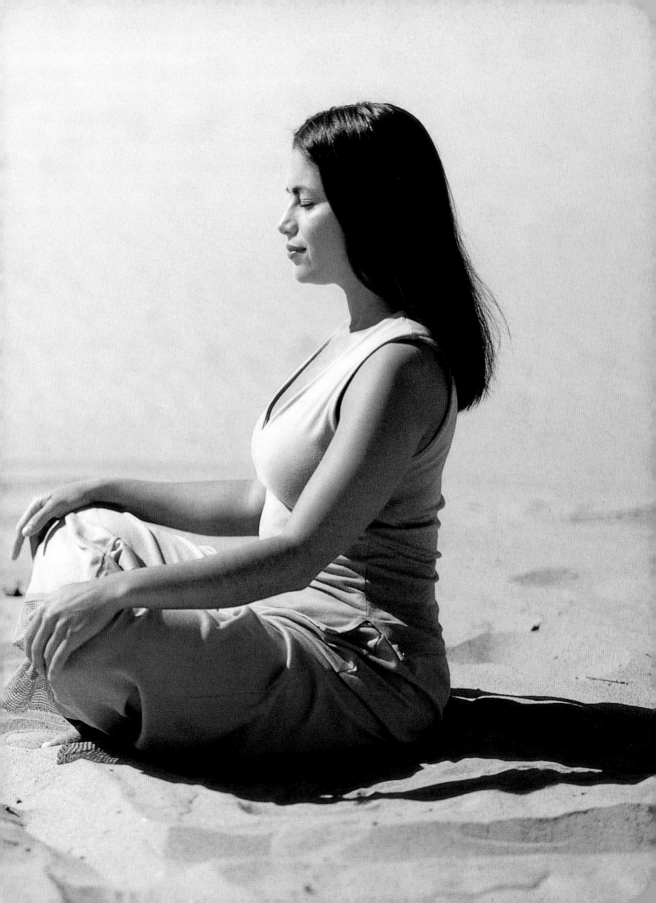

treatments and activities

Yoga

treatments and activities

Food and Nutrition

Romance and Partnering

glossary

acupressure A healing massage technique that uses thumb or fingertip pressure to stimulate acupuncture points.

acupuncture A 6,000-year-old Chinese healing tradition that involves placing needles into the skin at specific points to balance the flow of *chi* and treat illnesses.

antioxidant A molecule that suppresses various effects of oxidation and in particular free radicals, especially the short-lived, highly reactive oxygen types.

aromatherapy The skilled use of essential oils to promote physical, emotional, and spiritual wellbeing. The essential oils may be heated, dropped into baths, or applied (in a diluted form) to the skin.

aromatic oil See essential oil.

asana The Sanskrit term for a yoga pose. *Asanas* are designed to improve physical, spiritual, and emotional health.

astringent See *toner*.

Ayurveda The traditional medicine of India. This holistic health-care system teaches that each person has a core of peace and perfection—a natural state of wellbeing and happiness. Ayurvedic practices help people return to this natural state by balancing their life energies and helping them achieve harmony with the environment.

Bikram yoga A modern form of yoga that consists of 26 poses practiced in hot rooms to promote detoxification.

bromelain An enzyme that aids digestion. It's found in foods such as pineapple.

calorie A unit of measurement used in some countries to describe how much energy a food item has. Multiply calories by 4.186 for the equivalent in kilojoules.

carbohydrates Carbohydrates are essentially sugar and starch; when used as energy, they become fuel for our muscles and brain. They can be found in foods such as bread, grains, potatoes, apples, oranges, and candy.

carpal tunnel syndrome A condition in which the nerve in the wrist becomes compressed (often by repetitive motion) and causes weakness and pain.

carrier oil An inert oil (usually vegetable or mineral) used to hold or dilute more potent substances such as essential oils. A carrier oil is generally used to reduce the concentration of a substance, making it safe for use on the skin.

cellulite Subcutaneous fat with a pitted appearance, much like an orange peel.

chakra Translated as "wheel" in Sanskrit, a *chakra* is a point through which energy enters and leaves the body. Eastern traditions believe that the body has seven chakras, each associated with certain mental or emotional characteristics.

chi In Chinese medicine, *chi* is the vital life energy that flows through the body (and the universe). Chinese healers believe that blockages or deficiencies of chi are the root cause of disease.

cholesterol A waxy fat that comes both from the liver and from foods we eat, especially meat and dairy products. Nutritionists divide cholesterol into two groups: HDL cholesterol, which is considered "good," and LDL cholesterol, which is considered "bad," or unhealthful.

citronella oil An essential oil that is known for its bug-repelling properties.

collagen The main protein in connective tissue. Collagen lends skin its strength.
The degradation of collagen is a cause of the formation of wrinkles.

comedogenic Describes a substance that can cause or worsen pimples, blackheads, and whiteheads (to identify products intended to discourage these types of skin problems, look for the term *non-comedogenic* on product labels).

conditioner A substance designed to restore the healthy look of hair, which may have been damaged by excessive heat, chemical processes, or rough handling.

dietary fiber The bulky part of food (generally plants) that cannot be broken down by enzymes in the digestive system. Fiber helps move food through the intestines faster, and its consumption has been linked to decreased rates of cancer.

diffuser A device that distributes (often via heat) the aroma from an essential oil.

diuretic Any substance that increases the amount of urine the body produces.

elastin A protein that makes skin elastic.

ellagic acid A phytochemical with strong antioxidant and antibacterial properties. It's found in foods such as strawberries.

endocrine system The system of glands that produce various chemical secretions (hormones) that circulate, via the blood, throughout the body.

essential oil An oil that gives plants their characteristic odor. These oils are used for aromatherapy, as well as in perfumery.

exfoliant A grainy scrub agent designed to help clear skin of its residual dead cells.

exfoliate To scrub off dead skin cells.

fats Organic compounds that make up the most concentrated source of energy in food. *Total fat* measures all types of fat in a food. *Saturated fat* measures only the amount of a specific type of fat, which is the biggest dietary source of high LDL levels (or "bad" cholesterol).

free radicals Unstable molecules that have been linked to the degeneration of human biological functions. Free radicals are thought to contribute to disorders such as heart disease and cancer.

glutes The nickname for the *glutei maximi,* the muscles in the buttocks.

hamstrings The long muscles that run along the back of the thighs.

hatha yoga A form of yoga that combines postures and breathing exercises to balance the body's energies. The word *hatha* comes from the Sanskrit words *ha* (sun) and *tha* (moon); the goal of the practice is to unite and balance solar (energizing) and lunar (relaxing) energies.

heart chakra The "energy center" in the heart; this chakra is associated with love and generosity (see *chakra*).

heliotrope A plant with fragrant flowers ranging in color from violet to white.

kilojoule A unit of measurement used internationally to describe how much energy a food item has. Divide kilojoules by 4.186 for the equivalent in calories.

kosher salt A refined yet coarse-grained salt that contains no additives (it's called kosher because it is used to make meat kosher by drawing out the blood).

labyrinth A network of passages or paths, all leading to one central spot.

lactic acid A by-product of a process that delivers energy to muscles when they demand more oxygen than the blood can deliver. Lactic acid can cause a burning sensation during vigorous exercise.

loofah A rough sponge that is made from the dried pod of a gourd and is a good tool to use for exfoliating skin.

lymphatic system A network of spaces between body tissues and organs through which lymph (a pale fluid that has white blood cells in it) circulates.

melanin A naturally occurring dark pigment that is found in the skin or hair. When we're exposed to sunlight, our skin darkens because the skin produces more melanin.

meridian In Chinese medicine, a channel or path in the body through which energy (or *chi*) travels. Acupuncture points are located along the meridians; stimulating those points helps balance the flow of chi along that meridian.

metabolic waste The normal waste products that the body makes in the course of its day-to-day functioning.

moisturizer A substance or product that reduces moisture loss from the skin.

nadis Sometimes translated as "conduits," "nerves," or "vessels," Ayurvedic nadis—like Chinese meridians—are the channels through which life energy flows.

neroli oil Produced from the white blossoms of the bitter or Seville orange tree, neroli oil (also called orange blossom oil) exudes an aroma that aromatherapists say can help calm emotions, as well as help promote restful sleep.

neurotransmitter A substance that transmits impulses between nerve cells.

orrisroot Derived from the roots of iris plants, it is used as a fixative (or fragrance preservative) in perfumes and elsewhere.

osteoporosis A syndrome in which the bones become less dense, more brittle, and prone to breakage.

phenols A category of *phytochemicals,* including the compounds that make berries blue and eggplants violet. Phenols are potent antioxidants with anticlotting and anti-inflammatory properties.

phytochemicals Plant chemicals. Some *phytochemicals* have been reported to fight or protect against many diseases, ward off cell damage, stimulate the immune system, and aid the body's detoxification mechanisms.

Pilates A system of exercises developed by the German dancer and boxer Joseph Pilates in the 1920s. Pilates exercises strengthen and elongate muscles, thus improving posture and flexibility.

polyphenols A type of phenols found in substances such as wine, coffee, and tea. Polyphenols are potent antioxidants.

pores The openings to the sweat gland tubes on the surface of the skin. Sweat glands secrete perspiration and help regulate body temperature.

prana The Sanskrit word for life force.

pranayama Yogic breathing exercises designed to increase *prana,* or life force.

proteins Complex organic compounds made up of amino acids that supply the body with energy and enable functions such as building tissue. Food sources that are high in protein include meat, dairy products, grains, and legumes.

pumice stone A very light and porous volcanic rock that can be used to scrub off rough skin, especially on the feet.

quads (quadriceps) The muscles that run along the front of the thighs.

reflexology A type of massage that involves applying pressure to specific points on the hands and feet based on the belief that this pressure can benefit other body parts.

repetitive-stress injury An injury to cartilage, tendons, ligaments, nerves, or muscles that results from doing the same physical motion repeatedly.

Sanskrit An ancient language in India that is used in academia and religion—much like Latin is used in Western countries.

scrub A product designed to exfoliate dead skin cells that contains small granules.

self-tanning lotion A product containing dihydroxyacetone (DHA) that reacts with amino acids in the uppermost skin layers to trigger melanin-producing cells and make the skin look tanned.

Spleen 16 An acupressure point, at the base of the rib cage directly below each nipple, used to relieve indigestion, nausea, and abdominal cramps, and to balance the appetite and gastrointestinal system.

T-zone The forehead, nose, and chin on the human face, which tend to be oilier than other areas of the face.

tai chi An ancient Chinese fighting and healing tradition that consists of slow, graceful movements designed to balance and strengthen the body's *chi,* or energy.

terpenes A category of phytochemicals found in foods ranging from spinach to soy. Terpenes are powerful antioxidants.

thymus gland A ductless gland in the throat area that aids the immune system.

toner Also called astringent or freshener. A facial cleansing product that removes residual traces of make-up, oil, and other impurities. Toner has a refreshing and cooling action on the skin. It also can temporarily make pores look smaller.

yoga An ancient Indian system that combines *asanas* (physical poses) with *pranayama* (breathing) and meditation. The goal of yoga is to enhance physical, emotional, and spiritual health.

yogi One who practices yoga.

index

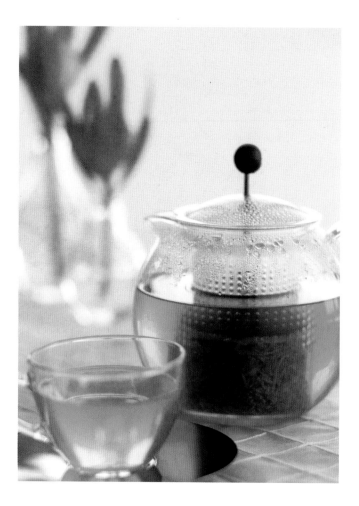

weldonowen

415 Jackson Street
San Francisco, CA 94111
www.weldonowen.com

President, CEO Terry Newell
VP, Sales Amy Kaneko
VP, Publisher Roger Shaw
Executive Editor Mariah Bear
Project Editor Elizabeth Dougherty
Assistant Editor Bridget Fitzgerald
Editorial Assistant Ian Cannon
Creative Director Kelly Booth
Senior Designer Meghan Hildebrand
Assistant Designer Sarah Edelstein
Production Director Chris Hemesath
Production Manager Michelle Duggan

Weldon Owen is a division of
BONNIER

Library of Congress Control Number
on file with the publisher

ISBN 978-1-61628-452-7

10 9 8 7 6 5 4 3 2 1
2013 2014 2015 2016

Printed in China by 1010 Printing

Weldon Owen would like to thank Barbara
Genetin for designing the chapter openers
and cover, Katharine Moore for
copyediting, Marisa Solis for proofreading,
and Andrew Joron for the index.

A version of this book was published in
2003 under the name The Body Care
Manual. That book could not have been
created without the invaluable
contributions of Creative Director
Emma Boys and Publications Manager
Justine Roddick.

Acknowledgements

All photographs courtesy of John Robbins, with the following exceptions:

Sheri Giblin 12, 26, 48, 80, 91, 108, 119, 121, 142, 149, 167, 203

Shutterstock Table of Contents, Introduction, Taking Care, 4, 14, 18, 23, 31 (sidebar), 33, 42, 45 (sidebar), 47, 65, 68 (sidebar), 73 (sidebar), 82, 85, 86, 89 (sidebar), 90, 92, 97, 98 (sidebar), 101, 102, 103, 104 (sidebar), 105 (sidebar), 106, 110, 112, 115, 129, 131, 135 (sidebar), 136, 141, 143, 151, 163, 164, 172 (sidebar), 176 (sidebar), 178, 185 (sidebar), 189, 192, 198, 201, 202, 203 (sidebar)

iStock 105